MicroRNAs in malignant tumors of the skin

Michael Sand

MicroRNAs in malignant tumors of the skin

First steps of tiny players in the skin to a new world of genomic medicine

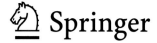 Springer

Priv.-Doz. Dr.med. Michael Sand
Bochum, Germany

ISBN 978-3-658-12793-0   ISBN 978-3-658-12794-7   (eBook)
DOI 10.1007/978-3-658-12794-7

Library of Congress Control Number: 2016939488

This Springer imprint is published by Springer Nature
The registered company is Springer Fachmedien Wiesbaden GmbH

Acknowledgments

I would first and foremost like to thank my clinical and scientific teacher, Professor Peter Altmeyer, for his support far above and beyond the norm, his excellent loyalty, and the unlimited access to all the needed resources of the clinic, which has fostered my personal and academic development to a great degree.

Special thanks goes to the Head of Dermatological Surgery, Professor Falk G. Bechara, for his unparalleled support in the development of scientific questioning and ideas, as well as for the education on performing operations, which I was able to gain in his department. As an academic teacher and as a friend, he has enabled the creation of this work with his extraordinary backing.

I would like to deeply thank Dr. Marina Skrygan, who stood by my side in cases of molecular-biological questions with impressive specialist knowledge under great personal involvement over the past years, and through this has contributed massively to the creation of this work.

I would like to thank my colleague Mr. Dimitrios Georgas for the excellent sample coordination in the Dermatological Surgery unit, and the Director of the Skin Tumor Center, Professor Thilo Gambichler for the extraordinary expert knowledge in statistical questioning and in the development of scientific questioning.

I would especially like to express my particular thanks to my mother and my brother, who have enabled this work through their patience and their encouragement in the past years.

Table of Contents

1   Introduction

In malignant tumors, uncontrolled cell replication occurs, which can be caused by a loss of function of tumor suppressor genes or the activation of oncogenes. These alterations have an immediate effect on the cell cycle. As a component of tumorigenesis, uncontrolled cell division manifests clinically as a malignant tumor. A number of studies have shown that the regulation of both tumor suppressor genes and tumor growth-promoting oncogenes is regulated by microRNAs (miRNAs) [1-3]. Whether miRNAs in skin tumors also assume a molecular-pathological role has not been investigated to any great extent and is the subject of this work.

1.1   MicroRNAs

MicroRNAs (miRNAs) are 17 to 23 nucleotides long, non-protein coding ribonucleic acids that play a fundamental role in post-transcriptional gene regulation [4-7]. Until approximately 20 years ago, the prevailing opinion was that only the protein-coding 1.5% of the approximately three billion base pairs of human DNA have a cellular function [8]. The remaining, non-coding components of DNA were falsely labeled "junk DNA" [9,10]. It was accepted that these large, non-protein-coding portions of the DNA were ballast, which humans had collected as part of their evolution. This hypothesis was disproven by the discovery of miRNA and the concept of RNA interference (RNAi) because it was shown that the non-coding areas of DNA also code miRNAs along with many other non-protein coding RNAs (ncRNAs), such as siRNA (small interfering RNA), piRNA (piwi-interacting RNA), snRNA (small nuclear RNA) and snoRNA (small nucleolar RNA) [4,11-14]. Through complementary base pairing between the bases of the miRNA and the target mRNA, there is translational inhibition, which significantly contributes to gene regulation [12,15-17]. A specific miRNA can have multiple target mRNAs, just as several miRNAs can also have the same target mRNA. miRNAs have been proven to exist in viruses and in plant, animal, and human cells [18-23]. The sequences of 2,042 human miRNAs were published in the current Version 19 (status as of August 2012) of the official miRNA database miRBase [24]. The list of described miRNAs is constantly growing, and current bioinformatic studies state that 30 to 60% of all human genes are regulated by miRNAs [25-27]. A multitude of important cellular processes, such as proliferation, differentiation, and apoptosis, are regulated by miRNAs [28-31].

1.2 MicroRNA maturity and function

miRNA coding sequences are localized both on introns and on exons of the DNA in the cell nucleus [32-34]. The overwhelming portion (80 to 87%) of the miRNA sequences are on the non-protein-coding introns [34]. miRNA maturation initially begins in the cell nucleus with the transcription of many kilobase-long primary miRNA transcripts (pri-miRNA), mainly through RNA polymerase II but also partially through RNA polymerase III (Fig. 1-1) [35-37]. The pri-miRNA created by this process has a characteristic stem-loop structure, a poly(A) tail at the 3' end and a 7-methylguanosine cap at the 5' end [38]. The pri-miRNA is split into multiple pre-miRNAs (precursor miRNAs) inside the cell nucleus through what is called the microprocessor complex [39]. The 500- to 650-kDa microprocessor complex consists of the RNase III Drosha and the double-stranded RNA-binding domain (dsRBD) DiGeorge syndrome critical region gene 8 (DGCR8, Pasha, **Pa**rtner of Dro**sha** in *Drosophila melanogaster* and *Caenorhabditis elegans*) [40-43]. DGCR8 has two binding locations for double-stranded RNA (dsRNA) and through them allows for the indirect binding of Drosha to the locations on the pri-miRNA that will be cut [44-47]. The stem-loop structure of the pri-miRNA consists of an approximately 33 base pair-long, double-stranded RNA (dsRNA) with a terminal contour with incomplete, imperfect complementarity and flanking short single strands of RNA (ssRNA, single-stranded RNA). DGCR8 recognizes the ssRNA/dsRNA transitions of the pri-miRNA [46]. Both RNase domains from Drosha cut 11 nucleotides (nt) away from the stem-loop base to these ssRNA/dsRNA crossing locations [48,49].

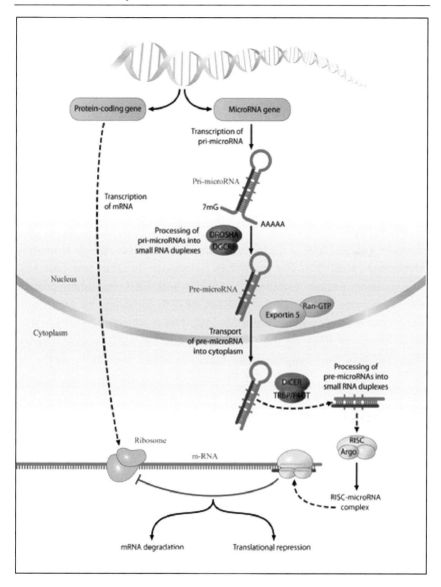

Fig. 1-1: MicroRNA maturity and post-transcriptional gene regulation (modified according to Chen [50]).

The pre-miRNAs resulting from this cutting process are 60-100-nt long and have a characteristic 2-3 nt-long overhang on 3' end [48]. While doing so, a terminal carboxy group of the DGCR8 regulates Drosha using a protein-protein interaction, and this leads to auto-regulation of the microprocessor complex [51]. Exportin-5 is a nuclear transport protein from the karyopherin family and binds the 2-3 nt-long overhang on the 3' end of the pre-miRNA [52-54]. In an energy-consuming process, the pre-miRNA is translocated from the cell nucleus into the cytosol [53-55]. In the cytosol, there is an additional essential maturity step. The RNase III enzyme Dicer cuts the pre-miRNA into an approximately 22 nt-long, double-stranded miRNA/miRNA* duplex with a 2 nt-long overhang at the 3' end [56-59]. MiRNA* designates the secondary strand that is complementary to the miRNA, which is usually dismantled [40,60,61]. The co-factors necessary for Dicer are TAR HIV RNA binding protein (TRBP or TARBP) and PKR activating protein (PACT) [62-65]. Dicer has two dsRNA binding locations, of which one recognizes thermodynamic instability [66]. The thermodynamically stable single strand of RNA on the 5' end becomes the miRNA main strand, while the less thermodynamically stable miRNA* secondary strand is usually dismantled [40,60,61,67]. The mature main miRNA strand is then loaded on the Argonaute-2 (AGO2) protein and forms the center of the RNA-induced silencing complex (RISC) [68-70]. Dicer, TRBP, PACT, and AGO2 form a RISC-loading complex (RLC), which simplifies the binding of the mature miRNA through Dicer to RISC [64,68,71]. RISC is the effector protein of the miRNA machinery. It is controlled by the miRNA and places itself like a molecular trestle on the target mRNA and prevents the ribosome from continuing to wander [72]. In doing so, the miRNA is bound to nucleotide positions two to seven. This area is called the "Seed Sequence" [73]. Depending on the degree of complementarity between miRNA, Seed Sequence, and the target miRNA, in some cases, there can be a complete complementarity to a cutting and a dismantling of the target mRNA or – more often in the case of incomplete but predominant complementarity – to a limited reading of the mRNA and, with it, a reduced translation in a protein by a ribosome [74,75]. An mRNA can be regulated in the process by different miRNAs, and an miRNA can, at the same time, regulate many different target mRNAs.

1.3   MicroRNA in oncology

Due to the many different cell regulatory activities of miRNA, there are strong indicators that miRNA could participate in the molecular pathogenesis of malignant tumors [76,77]. If one considers the recent history of the miRNAs, there are already indicators of this even in the first miRNAs described, in *C. elegans* and *Drosophila*. Given that, even very early on, the wide-ranging influence of miRNAs on the control of the cell cycle and on DNA repair mechanisms and, through this, on cell proliferation and apoptosis could be demonstrated, participation in malignant processes also appears very likely [78-80]. The sections coding for miRNAs are, moreover, usually near the gene sections mutated by malignant tumors [81]. Differences in the expression profiles of miRNAs from different malignant cells and the respective associated healthy controls have provided additional indicators regarding their participation in molecular pathogenesis [82-84]. This situation applies to malignant cells from cell cultures to the same extent as native tumor tissue. The two miRNAs hsa-miR-15a and hsa-miR-16-1 were the first to be described as dysregulated in a malignant tumor [85,86]. In the case of the chronic lymphocytic leukemia, CLL, in 68% of the cases, a deletion or reduced expression of these two miRNAs was shown, which promoted apoptosis in both by inhibiting the anti-apoptotic gene BCL2 [87,88]. This result demonstrates that miRNAs can regulate not just individual genes but also entire oncogenic signal cascades. The hsa-miR-17-92 cluster (also known as Oncomir-1) consists of the six miRNAs hsa-miR-17, hsa-miR-18a, hsa-miR-19a, hsa-miR-19b-1, hsa-miR-20a, and hsa-miR 92. It regulates the MYC gene on chromosome 8, which codes for the transcription factor c-Myc, a proto-oncogene that influences apoptosis [89,90]. Mutations in c-Myc are widespread in many different cancerous entities. An increased expression of hsa-miR-17-92 has been discovered in human B-cell lymphomas [91]. In a mouse model for B-cell lymphoma, the enhanced expression of hsa-miR-17-92, which for its part has an anti-apoptotic and an angiogenic effect, fostered a c-Myc-induced tumor [92-94].

An additional example for the participation of miRNAs in malignant processes is the regulation of the widespread proto-oncogene RAS, which is the product of a membrane-bound protein that promotes cell growth and proliferation. RAS is present in 15 to 30% of all malignant tumors. Inhibiting RAS leads to a tumor suppressor effect of miRNA let-7. A reduced expression of let-7 leads to an over-expression of RAS and, with it, enhanced tumor growth. In lung carcinomas, a reduced expression of let-7 and a correlation with clinical prognosis has been proven [95]. Therefore, let-7 is the first example of a tumor suppressor miRNA whose expression in the event of a lung carcinoma has informative value for prognosis [96]. A generally reduced expression of miRNAs was demonstrated by Lu et al. (2005) in 334 malignant tumors and tumor cell lines [82]. This work demonstrated a significantly reduced expression of miRNAs in a large number of different malignant tumors. Compared with highly differentiated tumors, slightly differentiated tumors demonstrate reduced miRNA expression. The reduced expression of miRNAs was associated with an increased tumor growth [97]. This result raises the question of whether the miRNA machinery and, in particular, the miRNA maturity enzyme in malignant tumors, are dysregulated. The miRNA maturity enzymes Dicer and Drosha have been proven to have an informative value for the prognosis of ovarian cancer patients [98]. Tumor samples with an increased expression of Dicer and Drosha were associated with a significantly longer survival time in patients. Similar results were described for neuroblastoma and breast cancer [99,100]. In contrast, other authors have reported an increased expression of the miRNA maturity enzyme with negative informative value for prognosis in cutaneous T-cell lymphoma and in soft tissue carcinoma [101,102]. In a mouse lung carcinoma model, a general reduction of miRNA expression was described when a Dicer deletion was present, which was accompanied by accelerated tumor growth, increased tumor load, and a reduced differentiation degree of the tumors [97]. Moreover, the reduced miRNA expression led to an activation of the proto-oncogenes RAS and c-Myc. Tumor suppressors were also regulated by miRNAs. In this way, p53 induced an activation of the pro-apoptotic miRNA hsa-miR-34 in the event of DNA damage [103,104].

In summary, it can be said that miRNAs represent a new group of central regulators of various signal transduction pathways with influence on growth and differentiation. To better understand the complex process of a malignant transformation, one must take the new group of miRNAs into account alongside the familiar concept of oncogenes and tumor suppressor genes. Their role in skin tumors has, until now, been minimally studied and is the subject of this work.

1.4 MicroRNA in skin tumors

The most frequent tumors in dermatology can be divided into epithelial skin tumors (also known as non-melanoma skin cancer, NMSC) and of melanocytic skin tumors.

Malignant melanoma

Malignant melanoma (MM) is a melanocytic, malignant tumor of the pigment-producing melanocytes that occurs mainly in the skin but can also occur in the eyes, ears, leptomeninges, the gastrointestinal tract, and in the oral and genital mucous membranes. The incidence rate in Germany is 21/100,000 inhabitants and has increased by 700% in the last 38 years [105]. The highest incidence rate described is for Australia and New Zealand, with 50 to 60/100,000 inhabitants. The current global incidence is, according to estimates from the WHO, approximately 130,000 new cases per year, with annual growth rates of 4 to 5%. A doubling of incidences is expected in the next 20 years for men and in the next 30 years for women, which makes the increase in incidence of MM greater than that in all other malignant neoplasias. Although malignant melanoma only comprises 4% of all skin cancer types, it is responsible for 80 to 90% of skin cancer-related deaths.

Malignant melanomas come from melanocytes, which are created in the neural crest of the neural ectoderm and travel in the form of melanoblasts as melanocyte precursors into the epidermis, the uvea, the meninges, and the ectodermal mucous membranes [106]. In the skin, the pigment melanin produced by the melanocytes forms protection against ultra-violet radiation in the *Stratum basale* (basal cell layer) of the epidermis, which will be discussed as the most important exogenetic factor under consideration of sensitivity to sun of the individual skin types for the formation of an MM [107]. While the exact wavelengths of the UV spectrum that are responsible for the formation of MM have not yet been definitively identified, it has already been shown that it is less the cumulative UV dose and rather the intermittent, high UV load of non-acclimated skin that is an important risk factor for the formation of MM [108]. This scenario is in agreement with the observation that people who work outdoors have a lower likelihood of developing an MM than people who work in protected spaces [109]. UV radiation in the form of sunlight, intermittent high UV load with non-acclimated skin, sunburns during childhood, and habitual use of tanning beds are external risk factors for the formation of an MM [110-112]. Skin type and hair color, age, number of melanocytic and dysplastic nevi, and the presence of ephelides (freckles) are among the individual phenotypical risk factors, as well as a diagnosis of MM in the personal medical history, a familial melanoma risk, or, in rare cases, genetic syndromes such as *Xeroderma pigmentosum,* in which the DNA's capacity for repair of regular, UV-dependent mutations is not present [107,113-116]. Malignant melanomas can exist in precursor versions (30 to 40%) and *de novo* (60 to 70%).

Alongside the more moderate locoregional aggressiveness, the inclination toward pronounced and early lymphogenes and hematogenic metastasis is to be emphasized. Due to this tendency to metastasize early and the poor response to chemotherapy, MM is the most dangerous skin tumor, which almost always ends in death if it has metastasized. Only surgical therapy in the early stage of an MM is a curative therapeutic option. Due to the currently limited treatment options in the advanced stage, an understanding of the molecular-pathological mechanism of melanoma genesis is important and is a basic prerequisite for improving the current therapy and developing new therapeutic options.

Molecular pathologically, various signal transduction pathways are known at the protein level, which participate in the pathogenesis of MM.

Although not all human miRNAs have been sequenced, some miRNAs are known to influence the signal transduction pathways involved in MM formation. One of the most important of these signal transduction pathways is presented in the following as an example:

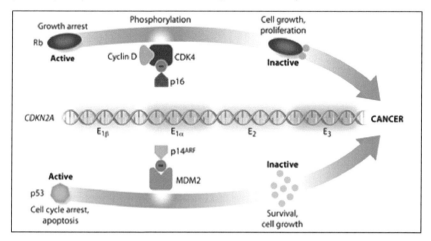

Fig. 1-2:   Cyclin-dependent kinase inhibitor 2A (CDKN2A) signal transduction pathway in melanoma (modified according to Nestle[117]).

The best-studied example is the high-risk allele cyclin-dependent kinase inhibitor 2A (CDKN2A), localized on chromosome 9, which above all plays a role in hereditary MMs [117]. CDKN2A codes the proteins p16 and p14-ARF, which inhibit the cell cycle. P16 competitively limits cyclin-dependent kinase 4 (CDK4). Together with cyclin D, CDK4 is in a position to deactivate the retinoblastoma protein (Rb) by phosphorylation; this event leads to an increased melanocytic proliferation. Usually, P16 inhibits the CDK4/cyclin–D-complex, so that the retinoblastoma protein remains active through the absence of the phosphorylation, and the cell cycle becomes inhibited.

p14-AFR, also coded by CDKN21, binds to the proto-oncogene MDM2, a negative regulator of p53, and inhibits the formation of p53 through MDM2. A mutation of CDKN2A contributes to the formation of an MM through a shorter melanocytic cell cycle. On the one hand, the result of a CDKN2A mutation is the inhibiting of the deactivation of Rb communicated through P16; on the other hand, the P14-ARF-communicated inhibition of the negative p53 regulator MDM2 is inhibited. In connection with this, Schulz *et al. (2008)* demonstrated that the miRNA hsa-miR-let7b leads to a reduced cyclin D and CDK4 expression [118]. For the first time, a direct influence of an miRNA on an established signal transduction pathway leading to the formation of the MM was demonstrated. Other inhibitions of gene expression communicated through miRNA could also play a role in the formation of the MM and are the subject of current studies [119].

Basal cell carcinoma

Basal cell carcinoma (BCC) is the most frequently occurring tumor in humans [120,121]. BCC involves a semi-malignant, slow growing but still locally infiltrating epithelial tumor that favors parts of the skin exposed to light. Clinically, we distinguish among nodular, sclerodermiform, superficial-multicentric, and pigmented BCCs. Large, ulcerating, growing BCCs are also designated *Ulcus rodens* and *Ulcus terebrans*. BCCs likely form from epidermal stem cells of the outer root sheath. Therefore, BCCs only occur on skin with hair follicles; palms of hands, soles of feet, and mucous membranes are unaffected. Metastasis is extremely rare and remains limited to reports of isolated cases [122-124]. Over the last 50 years, a steady increase in incidence of 3 to 8% per year has been observed. Risk factors described are as follows: UV radiation (particularly UV-B components 290 to 320 nm); geographic location; age; skin types I and II; male gender; and immunosuppression. Rare hereditary illnesses such as *Xeroderma pigmentosum*, Gorlin-Goltz Syndrome, oculo-cutaneous albinism, or *Epidermolysis bullosa* can be causes for an early development of BCC [125]. The gold standard treatment is a surgical therapy in the form of a micrographically controlled excision. If the lesion is not operable, alternative treatment options come under consideration in the form of cryotherapy or radiation. With superficial BCCs, photodynamic therapy is also possible. Although these very widespread tumor entities were already described in 1900 by Krompecher as "carcinoma epitheliale adenoides", the molecular pathogenesis is still not completely understood today [126]. BCCs usually occur sporadically and present molecular-pathological changes in the sense of activation of the so-called Sonic-Hedgehog signal transduction pathways [127,128]. Sonic-Hedgehog (SHH) is a signal molecule of the Hedgehog family, and binds to the Patched (PTCH1) receptor, which has a limiting effect on the Smoothened (SMOH) protein that is naturally present on the cell membrane [129]. SMOH limits an expression of the zinc finger transcription factor Gli1, which counteracts stoppage of the cell cycle and induces the development of hair follicle tumors [130-133]. Mutations of the PTCH1 receptor were demonstrated in 70% of the sporadic BCCs in the form of loss-of-function mutations [130,134,135]. In 10% of all BCCs, gain-of-function mutations of SMOH have been demonstrated. Whether there are changes in the expression of the components of the miRNA machinery or individual miRNAs in the BCC and whether this plays a role in tumor formation has only begun to be examined. Heffelfinger *et al.* (2012) compared the miRNA expression in nodules with that in infiltrative BCCs in a sequencing study based on miRBase 15 and described twenty miRNAs, which demonstrated a varying expression of these BCC subtypes on a significant level [136]. In another work, hsa-miR-203 was identified as a tumor suppressor in a mouse model, which was suppressed by activation of the molecular pathologically relevant SHH signal transduction pathway in BCC [137]. The study of the expression of the miRNA machinery and the description of miRNA expression profiles in BCC was performed as part of this work.

Cutaneous squamous cell carcinoma

Cutaneous squamous cell carcinoma (cSCC) is an epithelial tumor of malignant origin that can be dependent on both genetic and on exogenic factors. Similar to BCC, the UV component of sunlight is also the most important risk factor in cSCC. UV rays damage the DNA, resulting initially in the formation of intra-epithelial pre-cancerous lesions, the so-called actinic keratoses, which can lead to formation of cSCC. The face is affected in 90% of all cases [138]. In contrast to BCCs, which only very rarely metastasize, with cSCC, 20% of cases result in metastasis. If there is metastasis, the 5-year survival rate is 25 to 50%. In Germany, the incidence rate is at 40/100,000 inhabitants and can be up to 60/100,000 inhabitants in Australia due to the stronger UV load. Risk factors described are as follows: UV radiation; immunosuppression; heat; ionizing radiation; and exposure to arsenic and tar. cSCC is responsible for approximately 10 to 20% of skin cancer-related deaths. The gold standard therapy is a micrographically controlled excision. If there is metastasis, chemotherapies with cetuximab, cisplatin, fluoro-pyrimidine, bleomycin, and doxorubicin come into consideration [139,140].

From a molecular-pathological view, the most prominent and best-studied genetic change that was demonstrated early on in cSCC cells is a mutation in the p53 signal transduction pathway, which has a tumor-suppressing function in non-mutated, healthy keratinocytes (wild type) [129,130]. As in the formation of other malignant tumors, the Knudson hypothesis, which is the basis of the multi-mutation theory, also applies to cSCC [141,142]. While in cSCC cells there is a deletion of an allele of the p53 gene (first hit), there is a point mutation on the second allele (second hit). Consequently, there is a loss of the heterozygocity of the tumor suppressor gene p53. This situation results in a reduced apoptosis rate compared with wild type cells and, with it, a clonal growth of cSCC cells. Aneuploidy can be observed in 25 to 80% of cSCCs.

The previously described high-risk allele from hereditary MM, CDKN2A, and the tumor suppressor gene PTCH familiar from BCCs, which is important for the SHH signal transduction pathway, also show mutations in cSCC [130]. Little is known regarding the molecular-pathological participation of miRNAs in cSCC formation. Dziunycz et al. (2010) demonstrated an increased expression of hsa-miR-21 in vitro with UV-A-irradiated keratinocytes [143]. The tumor suppressor gene tropomyosin 1 (TPM1), programmed cell death 4 (PDCD4), reversion-inducing cysteine-rich protein with Kazal motifs (RECK), and tissue inhibitor of metalloproteinase 3 (Timp3) are partially inhibitors of matrix metalloproteinases (MMPs) and are expressed in a reduced form by hsa-miR-21 [144-146]. A reduced expression of RECK and Timp3 was present in squamous cell carcinoma of the lung, and there are indicators for a reduced TPM1 expression in the SCC of the tongue from mouse models [145,147-149]. A tumor-suppressive effect of hsa-miR-125b through the inhibition of MMP13 has been demonstrated [150]. To date, there have been no studies on the miRNA machinery and the determination of miRNA expression profiles in cSCC.

All presented signal transduction pathways are participants in the molecular pathogenesis of the respective skin tumor on the protein level. Despite only isolated first indications of the participation of miRNAs in the formation of the skin tumors described above, due to the ubiquitous function of miRNAs and their ability, depending on the mRNA target, to take on both a tumor suppressive and a tumor fostering role, the participation of miRNAs and the miRNA machinery in tumor formation is likely. A targeted, tumor-specific therapy that is in contrast to conventional chemotherapies could become possible in the future using synthetic miRNAs. The use of miRNA-based therapies in the case of malignant tumors is based on the restoration of the activity of tumor suppressing genes by using synthetic miRNA mimetics or the inhibition of oncogenes using synthetic miRNA antisense oligonucleotides, so-called antagomirs [151]. Although currently still in the experimental stage, the first pre-clinical successes have already been described in animal models in the miRNA-based treatment of lung and breast cancer as well as in glioblastomas, hepatocellular carcinoma, and pancreatic cancer [152-154]. In addition, with regard to an improvement of the response rates of a conventional chemotherapy, success has been described in other malignant tumors, such as ovarian cancer, with the use of miRNAs [155]. To contribute to the development of future therapies for malignant skin tumors, the expression of the most important components of the miRNA machinery and differentially expressed miRNAs in the three most frequently occurring skin tumors is studied in the work compiled here.

2 Objectives of this work

In this work, epithelial skin tumors (basal cell carcinoma and cutaneous squamous cell carcinoma) and malignant melanoma, as well as cutaneous melanoma metastases, are discussed.

In all three tumor entities, the expression of the most important components of the miRNA machinery (miRNA maturity, transport, and effect) are analyzed. Then, a characterization of differentially expressed miRNAs is made using the determination and analysis of miRNA expression profiles. The results of these studies should answer the following questions:

- Can significant differences in mRNA expression of the components of the miRNA machinery Dicer, Drosha, Argonaute-1, Argonaute-2, PACT, TARBP1, and TARBP2 be demonstrated using RT-PCR in basal cell carcinomas, cutaneous squamous cell carcinomas (cSCCs), and actinic keratoses (as pre-cancerous forms leading to cSCC)?

- Can significant differences of the Dicer expression be demonstrated at the protein level in malignant melanoma using immunohistochemical analysis?

- Can significant differences in mRNA expression of the components of the miRNA machinery Dicer, Drosha, Argonaute-1, Argonaute-2, PACT, TARBP1, TARBP2, MTDH, SND-1, and Exp-5 be demonstrated using RT-PCR in malignant melanoma and in cutaneous melanoma metastases?

- Can differentially expressed miRNAs be defined using microarray-based miRNA expression profiles in basal cell carcinomas, cutaneous squamous cell carcinomas, malignant melanomas, and cutaneous melanoma metastases?

3   Summary and discussion of this work

3.1   Studies on non-melanocytic, epithelial skin tumors

3.1.1   Expression of the miRNA maturity enzymes

SAND M, GAMBICHLER T, SKRYGAN M, SAND D, SCOLA N, ALTMEYER P, BECHARA FG (2010): Expression levels of the microRNA processing enzymes Drosha and dicer in epithelial skin cancer. Cancer Invest 28:649-653. [156]

The goal of this study was to determine the expression of the miRNA maturity enzymes Dicer and Drosha in actinic keratoses (AKs), cutaneous squamous cell carcinomas (cSCCs), and basal cell carcinomas (BCC) and to compare these expression levels with the expression in intra-individual and inter-individual healthy skin samples. This comparison should provide indicators of whether there is a change of the miRNA machinery as part of the carcinogenesis in epithelial skin tumors. For this purpose, first, intra-operative tumor samples and intra-individual and inter-individual healthy skin samples were collected through a 3-mm core biopsy. After RNA extraction, Dicer and Drosha expression was determined using a quantitative reverse transcription polymerase chain reaction (RT-PCR; Fig. 3-1 – 3-4). Both in the BCC and in the SCC group, a significantly ($p < 0.01$) increased Drosha expression compared with the inter-individual control group was shown (Tab. 3-1). The Dicer expression in the BCC group was significantly reduced compared with the inter-individual control group ($p < 0.05$). Dicer expression in the cSCC group was significantly higher compared with the intra-individual control group ($p < 0.05$), while compared with the inter-individual control group and for the cSCC and the AK group, no significant differences were found ($p > 0.05$). In the AK group, no significantly different expression compared with the intra- and the inter-individual control groups could be found for either Dicer or Drosha ($p > 0.05$).

In this work, a dysregulation of the mRNA expression of Drosha and Dicer in malignant epithelial skin tumors compared with a healthy control group has been demonstrated. Similar to a series of other tumors for which dysregulation of the miRNA has likewise been described, this could be an instance of a role the miRNA plays in the carcinogenesis of epithelial skin tumors. Like the Drosha expression in this study, similar observations have been made in cervical carcinoma [157]. There is no difference in the Drosha expression in either pre-malignant intra-epithelial lesions of the cervix or in the actinic keratoses as cSCC precursors. In cervical carcinoma, in contrast, an increased Drosha expression was observed, similar to cSCC. Similar to the expression of BCC in this study, a reduced expression of Dicer and for other tumors, such as ovarian cancer, was demonstrated [158,159]. Proof of the inhibition of the Dicer expression in BCC similar to the regulation of the Dicer expression in MM through the Sox-4 transcription factor is yet to be determined and is the subject of current research [160-162].

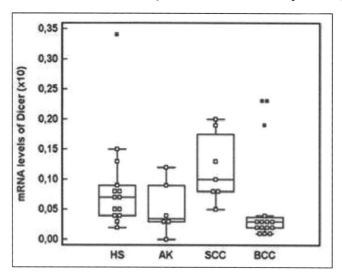

Fig. 3-1:   Box-whisker plot of normalized Dicer-mRNA expression (x10) in healthy subjects (HS), actinic keratoses (AK), squamous cell carcinomas (SCC), and basal cell carcinomas (BCC).

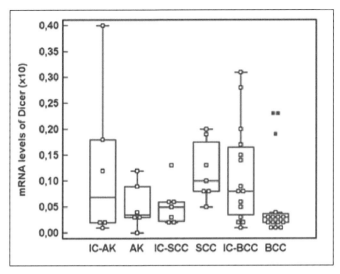

Fig. 3-2:   Box-whisker plot of normalized Dicer-mRNA expression (x10) in actinic keratoses (AK), squamous cell carcinomas (SCC), and basal cell carcinomas (BCC), as well as the corresponding intra-individual controls (IC-AK, IC-SCC, IC-BCC).

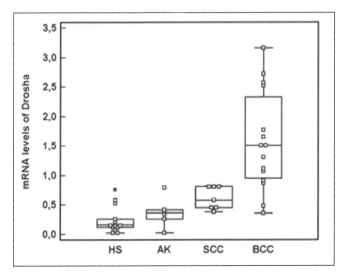

Fig. 3-3:   Box-whisker plot of normalized Drosha-mRNA expression in healthy subjects (HS), actinic keratoses (AK), squamous cell carcinomas (SCC), and basal cell carcinomas (BCC).

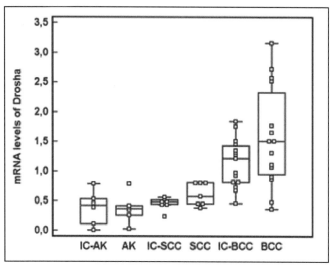

Fig. 3-4: Box-whisker plot of normalized Drosha -mRNA expression in actinic keratoses (AK), squamous cell carcinomas (SCC), and basal cell carcinomas (BCC), as well as the corresponding intra-individual controls (IC-AK, IC-SCC, IC-BCC).

Tab. 3-1: Data of the quantitative RT-PCR (qRT-PCR) of Dicer (x10) and Drosha (average ± standard deviation) in actinic keratoses (AK), squamous cell carcinomas (SCC), and basal cell carcinomas, healthy individuals (HS), and intra-individual (IC) controls of all tumor patients (IC-AK, IC-SCC, IC-BCC). (PS = primary sequence; RPL38 = human ribosomal protein R38; housekeeping gene; * = significant difference).

Parameters	Drosha HS control (a)	Drosha IC control (b)	Drosha AK (c)	Drosha SCC (d)	Drosha BCC (e)
qRT-PCR	0.25 ± 0.22 a versus b* a versus d* a versus e*	0.38 ± 0.29 (IC-AK) 0.46 ± 0.11 (IC-BCC) 1.15 ± 0.41 (IC-BCC)	0.37 ± 0.25	0.62 ± 0.2	1.57 ± 0.84

Tab. 3-1: (Continued)

Parameters	Dicer HS Control (a)	Dicer IC control (b)	Dicer AK (c)	Dicer SCC (d)	Dicer BCC (e)
qRT-PCR	0.089 ± 0.08 a versus e*	0.12 ± 0.15 (IC-AK) 0.05 ± 0.04 (IC-SCC) 0.11 ± 0.09 (IC-BCC) b versus d* b versus e*	0.05 ± 0.04	0.12 ± 0.06	0.06 ± 0.08

3.1.2   Expression of DGCR8 and the RISC components

SAND M, SKRYGAN M, GEORGAS D, ARENZ C, GAMBICHLER T, SAND D, ALTMEYER P, BECHARA FG (2012): Expression levels of the microRNA maturing microprocessor complex component DGCR8 and the RNA-induced silencing complex (RISC) components argonaute-1, argonaute-2, PACT, TARBP1, and TARBP2 in epithelial skin cancer. Mol Carcinog 51:916-922. [163]

The objective of this study was to determine the expression of the miRNA-mature component DGCR8 of the microprocessor complex and the RISC components Argonaute-1, Argonaute-2, PACT, TARBP1, and TARB2 in actinic keratoses (AK), cutaneous squamous cell carcinomas (cSCC), and basal cell carcinomas (BCC) and to compare them with the expression in inter-individual (HS) and intra-individual (IC) healthy skin samples. First, intra-operative tumor samples and intra-individual healthy skin samples were collected through a 3-mm core biopsy. After RNA extraction, the expression was determined using qRT-PCR. It demonstrated that the expression of Argonaute-1 (Fig. 3-5), Argonaute-2 (Fig. 3-5), DGCR8 (Fig. 3-6), PACT (Fig. 3-6) and TARBP1 (Fig. 3-7) in AK, cSCC, and BCC was significantly increased ($p < 0.05$; Tab. 3-2). The expression of TARBP2 (Fig. 3-7) showed no significant differences within the groups ($p > 0.05$). Both parts of the miRNA maturity machinery (DGCR8) and the miRNA effector RISC demonstrated a significant dysregulation ($p < 0.05$).

Argonaute proteins comprise the miRNA effector RISC. The over-expression of Argonaute-2 has already been demonstrated for squamous cell carcinoma in the head/throat area [164]. Because there is an over-expression of Dicer in cSCC as a part of RISC, an increased expression of other RISC components, such as Argonaute-2, was to be expected. DGCR8 is, alongside Drosha, a main component of the microprocessor complex, which is essential for Drosha function and miRNA maturity. With an over-expression of DGCR8, it can also be expected that Drosha will be over-expressed in both BCC and in cSCC [156]. While TARBP1 was likewise increasingly expressed, there was no significant difference in the expression of TARBP2. A possible cause for this could be no-loss-of-function mutations in TARBP2, which lead to a limitation of the miRNA function without influencing the expression of TARBP2 [165]. PACT likewise involves a RISC component, which also stimulates the protein kinase R (PKR) [166]. PKR stimulation favors apoptosis and was able to be demonstrated *in vitro* following UV irradiation of skin cells [167]. Based on the results of this study, a participation of the miRNA machinery in the carcinogenesis of epithelial skin tumors appears likely. Therefore, it appears sensible to describe specific, dysregulated miRNAs in additional studies as necessary.

Tab. 3-2: Data of the quantitative RT-PCR of Argonaute-1 and Argonaute-2 (average ± standard deviation) in actinic keratoses (AK), squamous cell carcinomas (SCC), and basal cell carcinomas, healthy inter-individuals (HS) and intra-individual (IC) controls of every tumor patient (IC-AK, IC-SCC, IC-BCC), * = significant difference.

Parameters	AGO1 HS control (a)	AGO1 IC Control (b)	AGO1 AK (c)	AGO1 SCC (d)	AGO1 BCC (e)
qRT-PCR	0.14 ± 0.05 a versus b (IC-AK)* a versus b (IC-SCC)* a versus b (IC-BCC)* a versus c* a versus d* a versus e*	0.9 ± 0.6 (IC-AK) 0.75 ± 0.57 (IC-SCC) 2.7 ± 1.4 (IC-BCC)	0.65 ± 0.55	0.64 ± 0.36	2.0 ± 1.53

Parameters	AGO2 HS control (a)	AGO2 IC Control (b)	AGO2 AK (c)	AGO2 SCC (d)	AGO2 BCC (e)
qRT-PCR	0.03 ± 0.01 a versus b (IC-AK)* a versus b (IC-SCC)* a versus b (IC-BCC)* a versus c* a versus d* a versus e*	0.07 ± 0.05 (IC-AK) 0.05 ± 0.02 (IC-SCC) 0.2 ± 0.08 (IC-BCC) b versus d*	0.06 ± 0.04	0.08 ± 0.02	0.39 ± 0.8

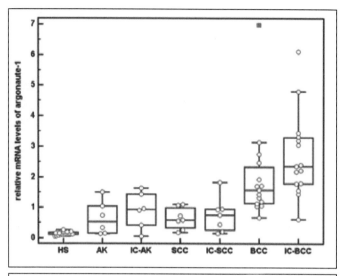

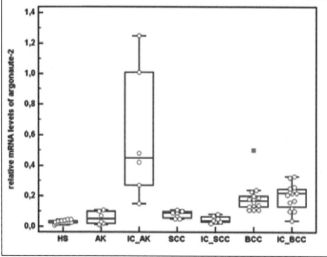

Fig. 3-5:   Box-whisker plot of the relative Argonaute-1 and Argonaute-2 mRNA
expression in actinic keratoses (AK), squamous cell carcinomas
(SCC), and basal cell carcinomas (BCC), and the corresponding
intra-individual controls (IC-AK, IC-SCC, IC-BCC), as well as in
healthy subjects (HS).

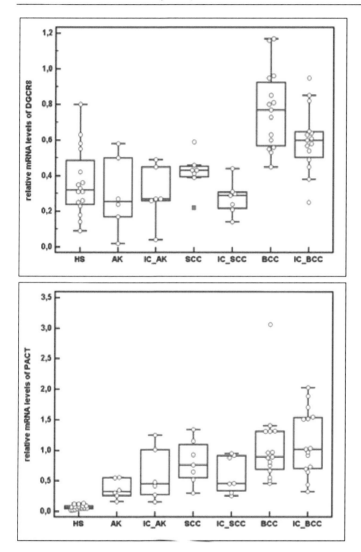

Fig. 3-6:   Box-whisker plot of the relative DGCR8 and PACT mRNA expression in actinic keratoses (AK), squamous cell carcinomas (SCC), and basal cell carcinomas (BCC), and the corresponding intra-individual controls (IC-AK, IC-SCC, IC-BCC), as well as in healthy subjects (HS).

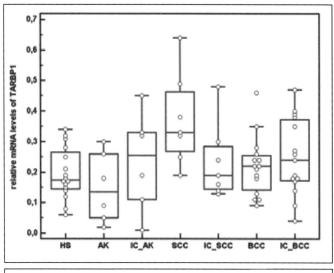

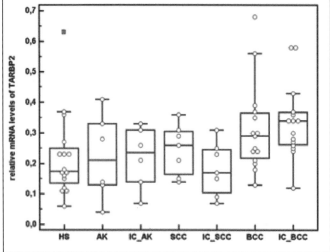

Fig. 3-7:   Box-whisker plot of the relative TARBP1 and TARBP2 mRNA
expression in actinic keratoses (AK), squamous cell carcinomas
(SCC), and basal cell carcinomas (BCC), and the corresponding
intra-individual controls (IC-AK, IC-SCC, IC-BCC), as well as in
healthy subjects (HS).

Tab. 3-3: Data of the quantitative RT-PCR of DGCR8, PACT, TARBP1, and TARBP2 (average ± standard deviation) in actinic keratoses (AK), squamous cell carcinomas (SCC), and basal cell carcinomas, healthy inter-individuals (HS) and intra-individual (IC) controls of every tumor patient (IC-AK, IC-SCC, IC-BCC), * = significant difference.

Parameters	DGCR8 HS control (a)	DGCR8 IC control (b)	DGCR8 AK (c)	DGCR8 SCC (d)	DGCR8 BCC (e)
RT-PCR	0.36 ± 0.19 a versus b (IC-BCC)* a versus e*	0.3 ± 0.16 (IC-AK) 0.28 ± 0.09 (IC-SCC) 0.6 ± 0.18 (IC-BCC) b versus d* b versus e*	0.3 ± 0.21	0.42 ± 0.11	0.77 ± 0.22

Parameters	PACT HS Control (a)	PACT IC Control (b)	PACT AK (c)	PACT SCC (d)	PACT BCC (e)
RT-PCR	0.07 ± 0.04 a versus b (IC-AK)* a versus b (IC-SCC)* a versus b (IC-BCC)* a versus c* a versus d* a versus e*	0.6 ± 0.44 (IC-AK) 0.6 ± 0.3 (IC-SCC) 1.13 ± 0.53 (IC-BCC)	0.36 ± 0.16	0.81 ± 0.36	1.06 ± 0.63

Tab. 3-3: (Continued)

Parameters	TARBP1 HS control (a)	TARBP1 IC control (b)	TARBP1 AK (c)	TARBP1 SCC (d)	TARBP1 BCC (e)
RT-PCR	0.2 ± 0.08 a versus d*	0.24 ± 0.16 (IC-AK) 0.23 ± 0.12 (IC-SCC) 0.25 ± 0.13 (IC-BCC) b versus c*	0.15 ± 0.11	0.37 ± 0.15	0.22 ± 0.1

Parameters	TARBP2 HS control (a)	TARBP2 IC control (b)	TARBP2 AK (c)	TARBP2 SCC (d)	TARBP2 BCC (e)
RT-PCR	0.22 ± 0.14 a versus b (IC-BCC)*	0.22 ± 0.1 (IC-AK) 0.18 ± 0.09 (IC-SCC) 0.34 ± 0.12 (IC-BCC)	0.22 ± 0.14	0.25 ± 0.08	0.32 ± 0.15

3.1.3 Expression profiles of microRNAs in basal cell carcinoma

SAND M, SKRYGAN M, SAND D, GEORGAS D, HAHN SA, GAMBICH-LER T, ALTMEYER P, BECHARA FG (2012): Expression of microRNAs in basal cell carcinoma. Br J Dermatol 167:847-855. [168]

The objective of this study was to create miRNA expression profiles of BCCs. During the operative removal of the BCCs, a biopsy was taken from the center of the tumor and from non-affected skin (intra-individual control). After successful RNA isolation from the samples, microarray-based miRNA expression profiles were created on an Agilent platform and analyzed (Fig. 3-9 and 3-10). As part of this process, per sample, 1,205 *homo sapiens* (hsa) miRNA candidates were screened. To validate the data acquired from the microarray, the expression of seven significantly dysregulated miRNAs were measured using TaqMan RT-PCR (Fig. 3-11).

In connection with the data validation and the bio-informatic data analysis, research was performed in the following databases: human miRNA-associated disease database HMDD (http://cmbi.bjmu.edu. cn/hmdd); miRNA database for miRNA functional annotations miRDB (http://mirdb.org/miRDB); Target Scan Human for prediction of miRNA targets (http://www.targetscan.org/), Mir2Disease database (http://mir2 disease.org/) [169]; miRò miRNA knowledge base (http://ferrolab.dmi. unict.it/miro); and miRBase (http://www.mirbase.org).

A total of 16 significantly up-regulated miRNAs (hsa-miR-17, miR-18a, hsa-miR-18b, hsa-miR-19b, hsa-miR-19b-1*, hsa-miR-93, hsa-miR-106b, hsa-miR-125a-5p, hsa-miR-130a, hsa-miR-181c, hsa-miR-181c*, hsa-miR-181d, hsa-miR-182, hsa-miR-455-3p, hsa-miR-455-5p, and hsa-miR-542-5p) and 10 significantly down-regulated (hsa-miR-29c, hsa-miR-29c*, hsa-miR-139-5p, hsa-miR-140-3p, hsa-miR-145, hsa-miR-378, hsa-miR-572, hsa-miR-638, hsa-miR-2861 and hsa-miR-3196) were described. The miRNA expression profiles strongly indicated that Oncomir-1 (miRNA cluster hsa-miR-17-92) participates in the pathogenesis of this epithelial skin tumor through the Sonic-Hedgehog signal transduction pathway known from the BCC. Hsa-miR-17, hsa-miR-18a, hsa-miR-18b (identical seed sequence with hsa-miR-18a) and hsa-miR-19b-1 (consisting of hsa-miR-19-b and hsa-miR-19b-1*) are significantly dysregulated components of Oncomir-1 [170].

Medulloblastoma, the most common brain tumor in children and simultaneously a clinical minor criterion of Gorlin-Goltz Syndrome (also known as basal cell nevus syndrome), is likewise associated with Oncomir-1 [171,172]. In addition, mutations of the Sonic-Hedgehog receptor protein patched homolog 1 (PTCH1) are found as a cause of Gorlin-Goltz Syndrome, as well as in 20% of cases of spontaneous medulloblastomas [128,173]. Participation of the miRNA cluster Oncomir-1 with BCC also appears likely. Alongside Oncomir-1, a series of additional miRNAs which are promising candidates for additional molecular-genetic studies were described as part of this study.

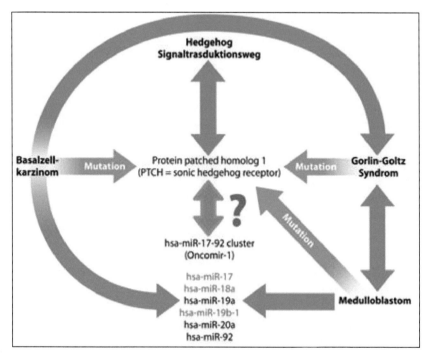

Fig. 3-8:   Mutations of the protein patched homolog 1 (PTCH1) show a possible association with Oncomir-1 (miRNA cluster hsa-miR-17-92) in basal cell carcinoma.

3.1.4   miRNA expression profiles in cutaneous squamous cell carcinomas

SAND M, SKRYGAN M, GEORGAS D, SAND D, HAHN SA, GAMBICHLER T, ALTMEYER P, BECHARA FG (2012): Microarray analysis of microRNA expression in cutaneous squamous cell carcinoma. J Dermatol Sci 68:119-126. [174]

cSCC is the second most frequently occurring epithelial tumor of the skin after BCC. To date, microRNA expression profiles have not been published for cSCC. The objective of this study, therefore, was to identify differentially expressed miRNAs.

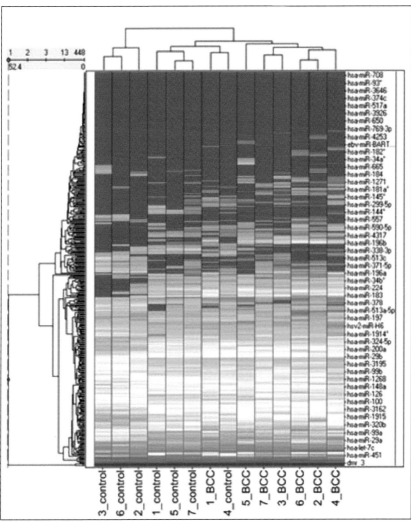

Fig. 3-9:   The miRNA expression cluster analysis shows a striking similarity to the expression data in the heat map with 448 filtered miRNAs. The color scale shows the log2 signal intensity, and runs from red (low intensity), through white (medium intensity), to blue (strong intensity). The dendrogram on the left side reflects the hierarchical similarity. The upper scale above the dendrogram indicates the number of clusters at different positions on the dendrogram. The lower scale is the similarity score for various positions in the dendrogram.

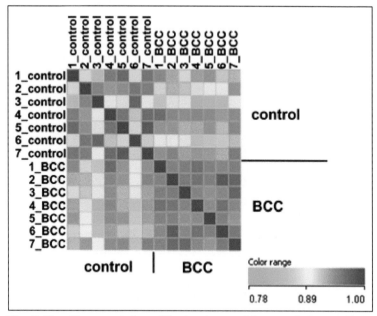

Fig. 3-10: Representation of the heat map of the correlation coefficient r of the miRNA expression profiles of basal cell carcinoma (BCC) and the control group acquired. The color scale on the right side shows the correlation of the samples and runs from green (medium correlation) to red (high correlation).

To do so, intra-operative cSCC biopsies and healthy skin biopsies (intra-individual control) were acquired. After RNA extraction, microarray-based miRNA expression profiles were created and analyzed (Fig. 3-12, 3-13). A validation of the microarray data was performed through a TaqMan qRT-PCR assay (Fig. 3-14). The data acquired in this way were then analyzed as part of research using the following databases: human miRNA-associated disease database HMDD (http://cmbi.bjmu.edu.cn/hmdd); miRNA database for miRNA functional annotations miRDB (http://mirdb.org/miRDB); Target Scan Human for prediction of miRNA targets (http://www.targetscan.org/); Mir2Disease database (http://mir2disease.org/) [169]; miRò miRNA knowledge base (http://ferrolab.dmi.unict.it/miro); and miRBase (http://www.mirbase.org).

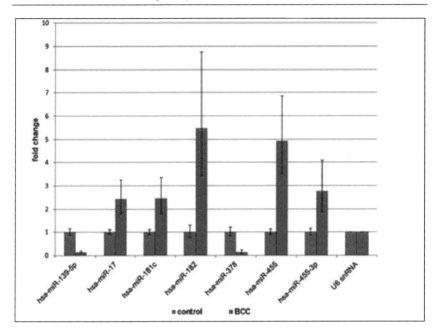

Fig. 3-11: The microarray results were confirmed using aqMan qRT-PCR based on up-regulated (hsa-miR-17, hsa-miR-181c, hsa-miR-455-3p, hsa-miR-455, hsa-miR-182) and down-regulated (hsa-miR-378, hsa-miR-195-5p) miRNAs.

Three significantly (p < 0.01) up-regulated (hsa-miR-135b, hsa-miR-424, hsa-miR-766) and six significantly (p < 0.01) down-regulated (hsa-miR-30a*, hsa-miR-378, hsa-miR-145, hsa-miR-140-3p, hsa-miR-30a, hsa-miR-26a) miRNAs were described. At a significance level of p < 0.05, 13 up-regulated and 18 down-regulated miRNAs were shown. Some of these miRNAs have already been studied in oncological studies. Hsa-miR-21 was also among the overexpressed miRNAs that are mentioned in the literature. An enhanced expression of hsa-miR-21 appeared *in vitro* after irradiation of keratinocytes with UV-A [143]. In addition, it was shown that the tumor suppressors reversion-inducing cysteine-rich protein with Kazal motifs (RECK) and tissue inhibitor of metalloproteinase 3 (Timp3), programmed cell death 4 (PDCD4) and tropomyosin 1 (TPM1) are expressed in a reduced form by hsa-miR-21 [144-146]. A reduced expression of RECK and Timp3 could be shown in squamous cell carcinomas of the lungs and for PDCD4 in a cSCC mouse model [145,147,148]. A reduced expression of TPM1 by has-miR-21 was present for the SCC of the tongue [149]. Hsa-miR-18a, which is a component of Oncomir-1 (hsa-miR-17-92 cluster), was among the over-expressed miRNAs [175]. In medulloblastoma, a connection could be demonstrated between Oncomir-1 and the Sonic-Hedgehog signal transduction pathway, which also plays an important role in cSCC [171,176]. In mice with mutated PTCH1, it was demonstrated that, in the event of an increased Oncomir-1 expression, there is an activation of the Sonic-Hedgehog signal transduction pathway and medulloblastoma development. In the case of breast cancer, there is an inverse relationship between the expression of hsa-miR-128 and interleukin 4 (IL-4). In oral SCC, a pro-apoptotic effect has been demonstrated for IL-4 [177,178]. Whether there is also a relationship between the overexpression of hsa-miR-128 and IL-4 expression cannot currently be answered. Tumor protein 53-induced nuclear protein 1 (TP53INP1), known as a tumor suppressor, is down-regulated by hsa-miR-130b, which is overexpressed in cSCC. An additional miRNA that is been overexpressed in cSCC is hsa-mir-133b. Similar to the results of our examination in cSCC, an overexpression of hsa-miR-133b has been demonstrated in oral SCC. In oral SCC cells, an overexpression of hsa-miR-133b and a dysregulation of the oncogene pyruvate kinase M2 (PKM2) dependent on hsa-miR-133b was demonstrated in vitro [179]. In our cSCC samples, hsa-miR-101 was significantly down-regulated. Myeloid cell leukemia-1 (Mcl-1) is a target gene of hsa-miR-101 and was already successfully inhibited by siRNA treatment in oral SCC cells in vitro [180]. Whether mcL-1 also plays a role in cSCC cannot currently be evaluated. Hsa-miR-204 was also down-regulated in cSCC. This had already been demonstrated for oral SCC. The tumor-suppressive effect of hsa-miR-204 has also been described for head-throat-SCC metastases [181]. The miRNAs described in this work are a suitable basis for additional studies as part of the carcinogenesis of cSCC.

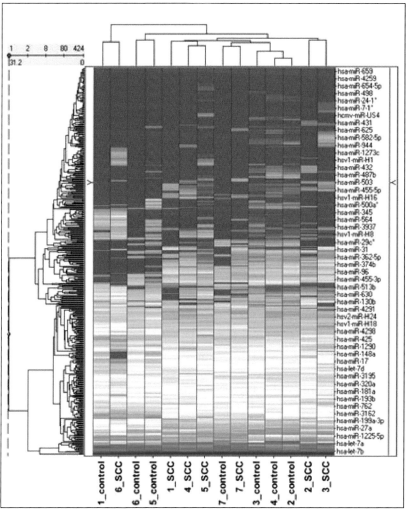

Fig. 3-12: Heat map of the cSCC and intra-individual control miRNA expression data with 424 filtered miRNAs. The cluster analysis shows, as in BCC, a high level of similarity to the expression data. The color scale reflects the log2 signal intensity, and runs from red (low intensity), through white (medium intensity), to blue (strong intensity). The dendrogram on the left side visualizes the hierarchical similarity. The upper scale above the dendrogram shows the number of clusters at different positions on the dendrogram. The lower scale shows the similarity score for various positions in the dendrogram.

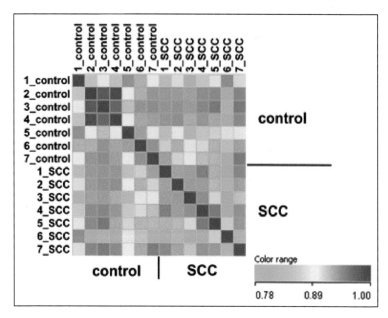

Fig. 3-13: Heat map of the correlation coefficient r of the miRNA expression profiles of the cSCC and the control group. The color scale on the right side shows the correlation of the samples and runs from green (medium correlation = 0.78) to red (high correlation = 1).

3.2   Examinations on malignant melanoma

3.2.1   *Expression of the miRNA maturity enzymes, transporters, and RISC components*

SAND M, SKRYGAN M, GEORGAS D, SAND D, GAMBICHLER T, ALTMEYER P, BECHARA FG (2012): The miRNA machinery in primary cutaneous malignant melanoma, cutaneous malignant melanoma metastases and benign melanocytic nevi. Cell Tissue Res 350:119-126. [182]

In this study, the following components of the miRNA machinery in primary cutaneous malignant melanoma (PCMM), in cutaneous

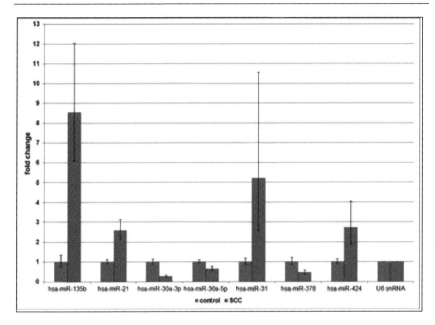

Fig. 3-14: Using TaqMan qRT-PCR, the microarray data were successfully validated. Both the significantly up-regulated (hsa-miR-135b, hsa-miR-424, hsa-miR-766) and six significantly down-regulated (hsa-miR-30a*, hsa-miR-378, hsa-miR-145, hsa-miR-140-3p, hsa-miR-30a, hsa-miR-26a) miRNAs were confirmed.

melanoma metastases (CMMM), and in benign melanocytic nevis (BMN) were determined using TaqMan qRT-PCR:

-   Dicer and Drosha (miRNA maturity enzymes)
-   Exportin-5 (Exp-5, pre-miRNA transport molecule)
-   DiGeorge syndrome critical region gene 8 (DGCR8; Drosha cofactor)
-   PKR activating protein (PACT; RISC component)
-   Argonaute-1 (RISC component)
-   Argonaute-2 (RISC component)
-   TAR HIV RNA binding protein 1 (TARBP1; RISC component)
-   TAR HIV RNA binding protein 2 (TARBP2; RISC component)
-   Metadherin (MTDH; RISC component)
-   Staphylococcal nuclease and tudor domain containing 1 (SND-1; RISC component)

The statistical evaluation resulted in Argonaute-1, TARBP2, and SND-1 having significantly higher expression in BMN than in PCMM ($p < 0.05$; Fig. 3-15 – 3-17). TARBP2 had significantly higher expression in CMMM than in PCMM ($p < 0.05$; Fig. 3-17), and SND-1 had significantly higher expression in CMMM than in PCMM and BMN ($p < 0.05$; Fig. 3-15). For Dicer, Drosha, DGCR8, EXP5, Argonaute-2, PACT, TARBP1, and MTDH, there were no significant differences within the groups ($p < 0.05$; Fig. 3-15 – 3-19). The results of the study show that the miRNA machinery components Argonaute-1, TARBP2, and SND-1 are significantly dysregulated in PCMM and CMMM in comparison to BMN ($p < 0.05$; Tab. 3-4).

A study based only on microarray data without RT-PCR verification produced the first indications for a reduced expression of Drosha and EXP5 in PCMM [183,184]. An over-expression of Dicer in PCMM was described in two other studies [185,186]. In our patient collective, we were able to only partially confirm the results published to date. Drosha and EXP5 showed a reduced expression in PCMM compared with BMN, but not at a significant level. In Dicer, there were no significant differences. In the study of the correlation of the individual components of the miRNA machinery, it was noticed that there is a participation of EXP5 in BMN in 4 of 9 correlation pairs. In PCMM, EXP5 does not participate in any correlation pair. This could indicate that the expression of EXP5 in PCMM is decoupled from the expression of other components of the miRNA machinery. Based on the data acquired here, a role of components of the miRNA machinery with regard to the malignant transformation in malignant melanoma appears probable and should be the subject of additional studies.

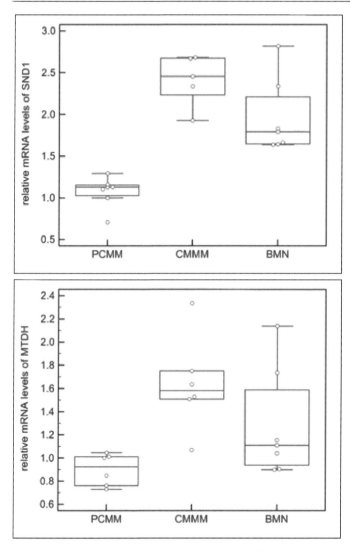

Fig. 3-15: Box-whisker plot of the relative mRNA expressions of the miRNA machinery components SND-1 and MTDH in PCMM, CMMM, and BMN.

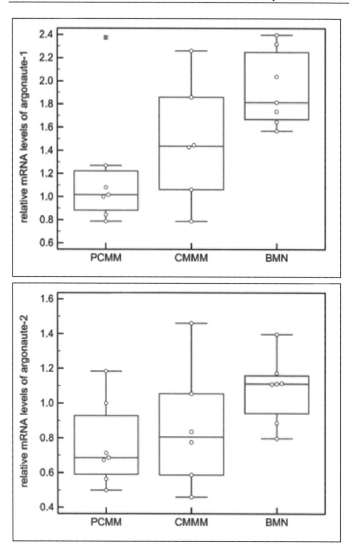

Fig. 3-16:   Box-whisker plot of the relative mRNA expressions of the miRNA machinery components Argonaute-1 and Argonaute-2 in PCMM, CMMM, and BMN.

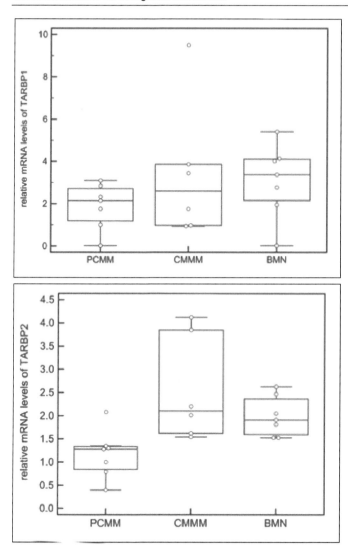

Fig. 3-17:   Box-whisker plot of the relative mRNA expressions of the miRNA machinery components TARBP1 and TARBP2 in PCMM, CMMM, and BMN.

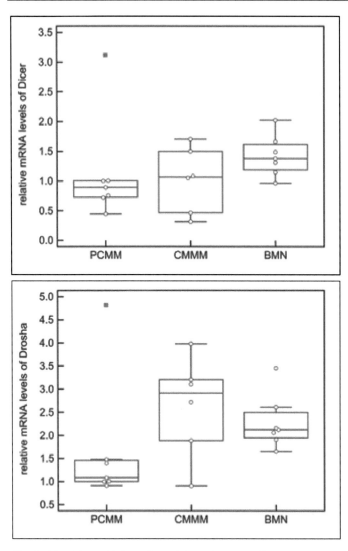

Fig. 3-18:   Box-whisker plot of the relative mRNA expressions of the miRNA machinery components Dicer and Drosha in PCMM, CMMM, and BMN.

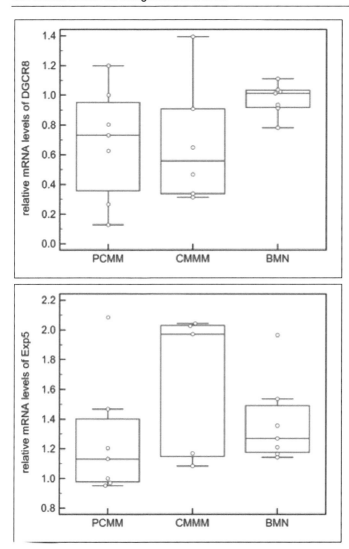

Fig. 3-19:   Box-whisker plot of the relative mRNA expressions of the miRNA machinery components DGCR8, Exp-5, and PACT in PCMM, CMMM, and BMN.

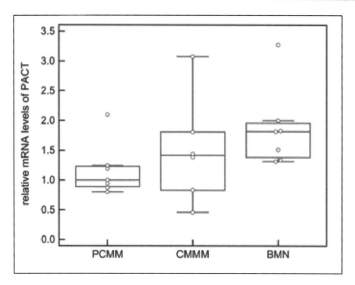

Fig. 3-19: (Continued)

3.2.2 Immunohistochemical study of the miRNA maturity

SAND M, GAMBICHLER T, SAND D, ALTMEYER P, STUECKER M, BECHARA FG (2011): Immunohistochemical expression patterns of the microRNA-processing enzyme Dicer in cutaneous malignant melanomas, benign melanocytic nevi and dysplastic melanocytic nevi. Eur J Dermatol 21:18-21. [185]

In this immunohistochemical study, the miRNA maturity enzyme Dicer was studied with regard to its expression at the protein level. Using immunohistochemical coloring, the Dicer antigen was colored in cutaneous malignant melanomas (CMM), benign melanocytic nevi (BMN), and dysplastic melanocytic nevi (DMN; Fig. 3-21). After semi-quantitative analysis, an expression index (EI) was determined, which considered the intensity of the immunohistochemical coloring and the overall surface of positive reactions in the two-dimensional histological paraffin cross-section of the components studied. The EI values were significantly higher in the CMM group than in the BMN group (p < 0.05).

Tab. 3-4:   Expression data of the quantitative TaqMan RT-PCR of Dicer, Drosha, DGCR8, Exp-5, Argonaute-1, Argonaute-2, PACT, TARBP1 and TARBPT, MTDH, and SND-1 (average ± standard deviation) in primary cutaneous malignant melanoma (a = PCMM), cutaneous melanoma metastases (b = CMMM), and benign melanocytic nevi (c = BMN), * = significant difference.

Parameters	PCMM (a)	CMMM (b)	BMN (c)
Dicer	1.13 ± 0.9	1.02 ± 0.55	1.42 ± 0.35
Drosha	1.67 ± 1.4	2.63 ± 1.09	2.28 ± 0.6
DGCR8	0.68 ± 0.38	0.68 ± 0.41	0.97 ± 0.11
Exp-5	1.26 ± 0.41	2.17 ± 1.33	1.38 ± 0.29
Argonaute-1	1.2 ± 0.54 a versus c*	1.47 ± 0.53	1.93 ± 0.33
Argonaute-2	0.76 ± 0.25	0.86 ± 0.36	1.08 ± 0.19
PACT	1.16 ± 0.44	1.5 ± 0.91	1.87 ± 0.67
TARBP1	1.89 ± 1.08	3.41 ± 3.23	3.1 ± 1.75
TARBP2	1.28 (0.40 ± 2.08) a versus b* a versus c*	2.11 (2.56 ± 4.19)	1.91 (1.52 ± 2.63)
MTDH	1.84 ± 2.5	1.64 ± 0.41	1.28 ± 0.47
SND-1	1.07 ± 0.18 a versus b* a versus c*	2.81 ± 1	1.96 ± 0.45

The EI differences between BMN and DMN as well as between CMM and DMN were not significant ($p < 0.05$). A significant correlation of the Breslow tumor thickness and Dicer-EI ($r = 0.84$, $p = 0.022$) was observed for CMM (Fig. 3-20). In all three groups studied, a positive Dicer coloration was observed in the epidermis, particularly in the melanocytes. This result was more strongly pronounced in melanoma cells than in benign melanocytes. After significant dysregulation of the miRNA expression had been determined using miRNA expression profiles in cutaneous melanoma, the results of this study indicated that changes in the miRNA maturity machinery also exist in cutaneous melanoma. Dicer is an essential enzyme for miRNA maturity and the orderly embryonic development of the skin [187]. The epidermis has an ectodermal origin, while the dermis has a mesodermal origin. Differing levels of metabolic activity of both embryonically distinctive parts of the skin could be a cause for the increased epidermal Dicer expression. The observation that malignant melanocytes show a stronger color in PCMM than melanocytes in BMN could be interpreted as an additional indication of a participation of the miRNA machinery on the molecular pathology of the PCMM. Additional studies are necessary to more closely evaluate the role that possible dysregulation of proteins from the miRNA maturity machinery other than Dicer also plays in cutaneous melanoma.

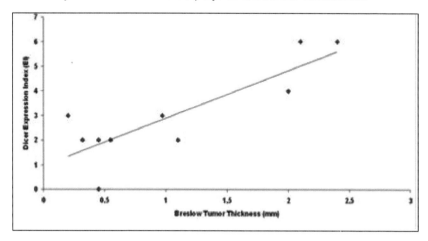

Fig. 3-20: Correlation of Breslow tumor thickness and Dicer expression (r = 0.84, p = 0.022).

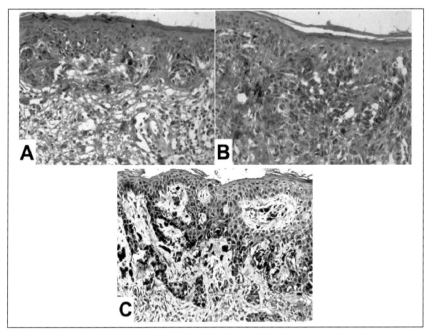

Fig. 3-21: Immunohistochemical coloring with an anti-Dicer antibody and Fast Red (chromogen) with dysplastic melanocytic nevi (A), malignant melanoma (B), and benign nevis (C) (400x magnification).

3.2.3   miRNA expression profiles in melanoma

SAND M, SKRYGAN M, SAND D, GEORGAS D, GAMBICHLER T, HAHN SA, ALTMEYER P, BECHARA FG (2013): Comparative microarray analysis of microRNA expression profiles in primary cutaneous malignant melanoma, cutaneous malignant melanoma metastases, and benign melanocytic nevi.
Cell Tissue Res 351:85-98. [188]

In this study, miRNA expression profiles of primary cutaneous malignant melanomas (PCMM), cutaneous malignant melanoma metastases (CMMM), and benign melanocytic nevi (BMN) were created. To do so, biopsies were obtained intra-operatively during the excision of the tumors. After RNA extraction, miRNA expression profiles were created using microarray and analyzed (Fig. 3-22, 3-23). To validate the data, a TaqMan RT-PCR of five significantly up-regulated and down-regulated miRNAs was performed (Fig. 3-24). In connection with the data validation and the bio-informatic data analysis, research was performed in the following databases: human miRNA-associated disease database HMDD (http://cmbi.bjmu.edu.cn/hmdd); miRNA database for miRNA functional annotations miRDB (http://mirdb.org/miRDB); Mir2Disease database (http://www.mir2disease.org/); and the Melanoma Molecular Map Project (http://www.mmmp.org/MMMP/). The miRNA expression profiles were also compared with profiles from older versions of the miRBase database. In doing so, 19 miRNA sequences not previously connected with melanoma were identified. The miRNAs has-miR-22, hsa-miR-130hashsa-miR-146hasp, hsa-has-223, hshasiR-301ahassa-miR-484, hsa-miR-663, hsa-miR-720, hsa-miR-1260, hsa-miR-1274 hashsa-miR-127has hsa-miR-3663-3p, hsa-miR-4281, and hsa-miR-4286 were significanhas up-regulhasd, whilhassa-miR-24-1*, hsa-miR-26a,hasa-miR-4291, hsa-miR-4317, and hsa-miR-4324 were down-regulated. The function and the expression behavior of the previously described miRNAs had largely not yet been described in connection with malignant tumors. In the following, the function of those miRNAs that were not previously connected with PCMM in the literature is presented. For pancrhasic cancer, an over-expression of hsa-miR-301a and the resulting activation of the nuclear transcription factor NF-κB were described [189]. Hsa-miR-301a inhibits the NF-κB expression-inhibiting factor Nκrf. For PCMM, an increased expression of NF-κB has already been described [190]. Whether the increased expresshas of NF-κB in PCMM is also regulated by hsa-miR-301a canhas currently be stated.

One target gene of hsa-miR-130b is the tumor suppressor tumor-protein-p53-inducible nuclear protein 1 (TP53INP1) [191]. In PCMM, a reduced concentration of TP53INP1 has already been demonstrated [192,193].

Hsa-miR-146b-5p, overexpressed in this patient collective, shows interactions with twhasolecular-pathologically relevant genes in PCMM. Hsa-miR-146b-5p reduces the expression of the epidermal growth factor receptors (EGFR) and mothers against decapentaplegic homolog 4

(SMAD4). SMAD4 is an important part of the TGF-beta signal transduction cascade, which demonstrates properties in PCMM that promote the formation of multiple tumors [194]. EGFR was overexpressed in PCMM cell lines and influences the metastasis of PCMM [195]. hsa-miR-26a shows a rhasced expression in the collective. The target gene for hsa-miR-26a is enhancer of zeste homolog 2 (EZH2), a cell cycle-regulating and transcription-limiting gene. EZH2 suppresses the expression of p21 (also known as cyclin-dependent kinase inhibitor 1 or CDK inhibitor 1), which suppresses tumor growth when the cell cycle is stopped [196-198]. No statements on the possible function of the remainder of the differentiahas exprehasd miRNAhasescribehasn this hasdy (up-hasulated: has-miR-22, has-miR-223,hasa-miR-484, has-miR-663hassa-miR-720, hsa-miR-1260hassa-miR-12has, hsa-mihas274b, hsa-mhas3663-3p, hsa-miR-4281, hsa-miR-4286; down-regulated: hsa-miR-24-1*, hsa-miR-4291, hsa-miR-4317 and hsa-miR-4324) can be made at this time; no tumor-relevant function has yet been attributed to them. The previously presented miRNAs are highly promising, new miRNA candidates for additional studies of their possible role in malignant melanoma. A software-supported analysis with a bio-informatic expert system, such as Ingenuity® Pathways Analysis (IPA) (Ingenuity Systems, Redwood, USA), could allow for new points of approach for the study of affected signal transduction pathways and miRNA target genes in the future [199].

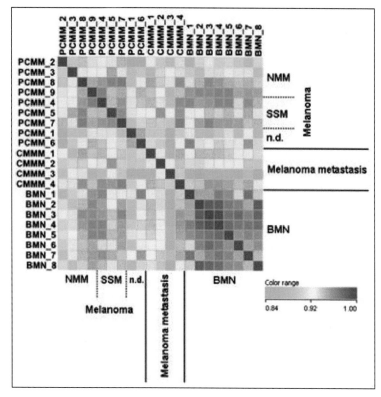

Fig. 3-22: Heat map of the correlation coefficient r of the miRNA expression profiles of the PCMM, CMMM, and BMN. The color scale in the lower right corner shows the correlation of the miRNA expression profiles of the respective samples among each other and runs from green (medium correlation = 0.84) to red (high correlation = 1).

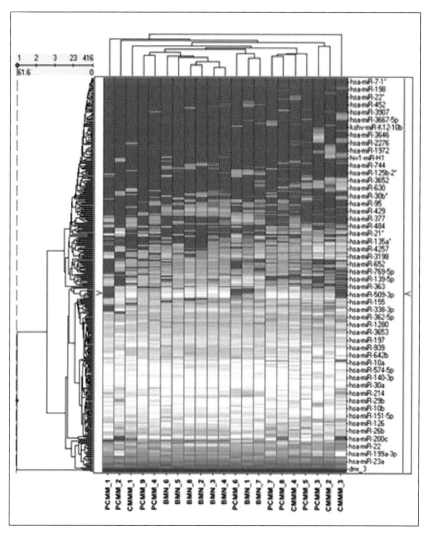

Fig. 3-23: Heat map of the miRNA expression data for PCMM, CMMM, and BMN. The cluster analysis shows a homogeneous pattern of the expression data. The color scale reflects the log2 signal intensity, and runs from red (low intensity), through white (medium intensity), to blue (strong intensity). The dendrogram in the upper left corner visualizes the hierarchical similarity. Above the dendrogram, the number of clusters at different positions on the dendrogram is shown.

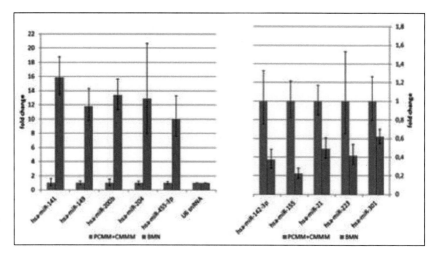

Fig. 3-24: The successful validation of the miRNA expressiohasrofileshas-
tained hasng the mhasoarray hasulted from a TaqMan qRT-PCR of
significantly downhasgulatehashsa-miR-141, hsa-miR-149, hsa-
miR-20has hsa-miR-204, hsa-miR-455-3p) and significantly up-
regulated miRNAs (hsa-miR-21, hsa-miR-142-3p, hsa-miR-155,
hsa-miR-223, hsa-miR-301a).

4 Closing remarks

The discovery of miRNAs and their functions has changed the understanding of the molecular pathology of a number of illnesses [4]. Due to their oncogenic and tumor-suppressive effects, the miRNAs in malignant tumors are particularly suited for the study of dysregulations [200-202].

In the work compiled here, first, the role of miRNAs in malignant skin tumors was described. In malignant melanoma, in cutaneous squamous cell carcinoma, and in basal cell carcinoma, dysregulated components of the miRNA machinery were characterized [156,163,182]. Using qRT-PCR, significant differences in the mRNA expression of Drosha, Argonaute-1, Argonaute-2, DGCR8, PACT, and TARBP1 could be demonstrated in BCC [156,163]. This likewise applies in cSCC for Dicer, Drosha, Argonaute-1, Argonaute-2, DGCR8, PACT, and TARBP1, as well as in actinic keratoses for Argonaute-1, Argonaute-2 DGCR8, PACT, and TARBP1 [156,163]. The mRNA expression of Argonaute-1, TARBP2, and SND-1 were significantly different in PCMM and CMMM [203]. Using immunohistochemical analysis, significant differences of the Dicer expression could be demonstrated at the protein level [185].

In connection with the mRNA expression studies of components of the miRNA machinery, miRNA expression profiles of PCMM, CMMM, cSCC, and BCC were created as part of a microarray-based study [168,174,188,204]. In doing so, altogether, 54 differehasally ehasessed mihass could be hasntifiedhasr PCMM ahasfor bothasSCC andhasC epithhasal tumorhas

In PCMM has CMMM, 14hasRNAs (hsa-mhas22, hsa-has-130b, hsa-miR-146b-5p, hsa-miR-223, hsa-miR-301a, hsa-mihas84, hsa-mhas663, hshasiR-720, has-miR-1260, hsa-miR-1274a, hsa-miR-1274b, hsa-miR-3663-3p, hsa-miR-4281, hsa-miR-4286) were up-regulated, and five were down-regulated (hsa-miR-24-1*, hsa-miR-26a, hsa-miR-4291, hsa-miR-4317, hsa-miR-4324) [188].

In BCC, thehaswere 16has-regulatedhasRNAS (hsa-miR-17, hsa-miR-18a, hsa-miR-18b, has-miR-19hashsa-miR-has-1*, hsa-miR-93, hsa-miR-106b, hsa-miR-1has-5p, hshasiR-130ahassa-miR-181hashsa-miR-181c*, hsa-miR-181d, hsa-miR-182, hsa-miR-455-3p, hsa-miR-455-5p and hsa-miR-542-5p) and 10 down-regulated (hsa-miR-29c, hsa-miR-29c*, hsa-miR-139-5p, hsa-miR-140-3p, hsa-miR-145, hsa-miR-378, hsa-miR-572, hsa-miR-638, hsa-miR-2861, hsa-miR-3196) [168].

In cSCC, three miRNAs were up-regulated (hsa-miR-135b, hsa-miR-424 and hsa-miR-766), and six were down-regulated (hsa-miR-30a*, hsa-miR-378, hsa-miR-145, hsa-miR-140-3p, hsa-miR-30a, hsa-miR-26a) [174].

The miRNA expression data obtained in this way make a contribution to identifying the miRNAs that participate in malignant skin tumors and are useful for the bioinformatic analysis of the metabolic pathways that participate in tumor diseases. In addition, they are a starting point for functional studies, which examine the effects of individually dysregulated miRNAs on tumor cells. The fact that it is possible to transfect synthetic miRNAs (miRNA mimics) into a cell or to bind individual miRNAs and withdraw them from a cellular function using antagomirs, which can be made complementary to a specific miRNA, particularly gives hope to future miRNA-based therapies [3,205-207]. In conclusion, through the studies presented here, there are significant indicators of a participation of miRNAs on the skin tumors studied here and makes additional studies in this new field of molecular dermatology appear promising.

5 Paper 1: Expression levels of the microRNA processing enzymes Drosha and Dicer in epithelial skin cancer[*]

5.1 Introduction

Micro-RNAs (miRNAs) are small, endogenous molecules between 21 to 27 nucleotides in length, capable of post-transcriptional gene silencing. According to the miRNA database (miRBase), 695 different human miRNAs have been described to date [1] and are thought to play important roles in the post-transcriptional regulation of up to 30% of all human genes. Both the intranuclear miRNA-processing enzyme Drosha and the extranuclear microRNA-processing enzyme Dicer play pivotal roles in the maturation of miRNAs [2]. Drosha is an RNase III endonuclease essential for the initial stages of miRNA biogenesis, cleaving pri-miRNAs (consisting of a hairpin stem, a terminal loop, and 5` and 3` single-stranded RNA extensions) to pre-miRNAs (60-70 nucleotide stem-loop structures). Once Exportin 5 transports pre-miRNAs to the cytoplasm, they are further cleaved by yet another RNase III enzyme called Dicer [3]. Dicer cuts the pre-miRNA at a predetermined distance from the 3´ end, resulting in short fragments or mature miRNA strands [4], which are then incorporated into the RNA-induced silencing complex (RISC). RISC is capable of modulating gene expression resulting in a variety of effects in the host cell, which is the subject of the current investigation [5].

Several miRNAs have recently been linked to tumorigenesis in many types of malignant tumors. miRNA expression profiles display both up- and/or downregulation in different human cancers, indicating that dysregulation of miRNA expression may be involved in carcinogenesis [6]. However, there has been limited research linking miRNAs to epithelial skin cancer. In this pilot study, we therefore investigated the expression levels of the miRNA processing enzymes Dicer and Drosha in basal cell carcinomas, squamous cell carcinomas, and actinic

---

[*] Co-authors: Thilo Gambichler M.D., Marina Skrygan Ph.D., Daniel Sand B.S., Peter Altmeyer M.D., Falk G. Bechara M.D.

keratoses (premalignant epithelial skin lesions), comparing expression levels from non-lesional skin samples (intraindividual controls) as well as from a healthy control group.

5.2   Materials and Methods

This prospective pilot study was initiated in a section of dermatologic surgery at an academic university hospital and was conducted within the framework of the declaration of Helsinki. Informed consent was obtained from all study subjects, and the study was approved by the Ethical Review Board of the Ruhr-University Bochum, Germany (registration number: 3265-08, ClinicalTrials.gov Identifier: NCT00849914).

5.2.1   Subjects

A total of 28 patients (10 females, 18 males; median age: 69.9 years) with a single type of premalignant skin lesion (6 actinic keratoses) or epithelial skin cancer (7 squamous cell carcinomas, 15 basal cell carcinomas) were enrolled in the study. Skin tumors were excised by scalpel under local anesthesia. Specimens were harvested with a 3-mm punch biopsy from tumor centers. Non-lesional control specimens were harvested from an adjacent healthy skin site near the tumor border (intraindividual controls). Additionally, a group of 14 healthy subjects (9 females, 5 males; median age: 68.4 years) were included as a second control group.

5.2.2   RNA isolation and real-time RT-PCR

Total cellular RNA was isolated from skin tissue samples using the RNeasy Lipid Tissue Kit (Qiagen, Chatsworth, CA, USA) following the manufacturer's protocol. Quantitative analysis was performed by real-time RT-PCR using the *Power*SYBR® Green PCR Master Mix and StepOne™ Real-Time PCR System (Applied Biosystems, Foster City, CA, USA). Primer Express software (PE Applied Biosystems, Foster City, CA, USA) was used to design PCR primers for Drosha, Dicer and the RPL38 housekeeping gene. Primers were produced by the custom oligonucleotide synthesis service TIB Molbiol (Berlin, Germany). The comparative

Δ-ΔC_t method was used as previously described by Livak and Schmittgen [6]. Relative amounts of target mRNA in test samples were calculated and normalized to the corresponding RPL38 mRNA transcript levels in each skin sample. To better illustrate mRNA quantities, the ΔC_t values (logarithms) were re-transformed, and Dicer expression data was multiplied by a factor of 10.

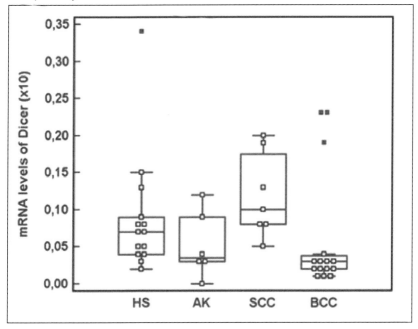

Fig. 5-1: Multiple comparison Box and Whisker diagram showing Dicer mRNA expression (x10) in healthy subjects (HS), actinic keratoses (AK), squamous cell carcinomas (SCC), and basal cell carcinomas (BCC).

5.2.3 Statistical analyses

Data analysis was performed using Med-Calc software (Mariakerke, Belgium). The null hypothesis was based on the assumption that there was no difference between Dicer and Drosha expression levels in SCC, BCC and AK specimens compared to healthy controls. Data distribution was assessed by the Kolmogorov-Smirnov test. In cases of non-normal distributions (such as for Dicer in the BCC group), data were analyzed by the Mann-Whitney test for independent samples and the Wilcoxon test for dependent samples. In cases of normal distributions (all other sample groups), data were analyzed by two-sided unpaired t-tests to compare tumor groups with healthy controls. For comparison of the tumor group and intraindividual controls, data were assessed by two-sided paired t-tests. All results were expressed as means ± standard deviation (SD) with statistical significance set at 5% (two-sided).

5.3   Results

Dicer expression levels in BCC samples were significantly lower compared to healthy controls ($p < 0.05$) (Fig. 5-1). The mean Dicer expression level was also lower compared to intraindividual controls, but was not statistically significant ($p > 0.05$). Dicer levels in both the SCC and AK groups were not significantly different compared to healthy controls ($p > 0.05$) (Fig. 5-1). However, the SCC group did show significantly higher Dicer expression levels compared to intraindividual controls ($p < 0.05$) (Fig. 5-2).

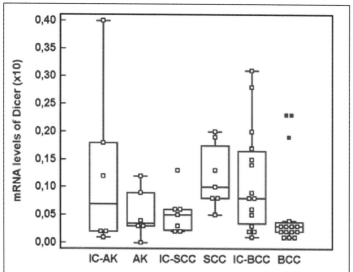

Fig. 5-2:   Multiple comparison Box and Whisker diagram showing Dicer mRNA expression (×10) in actinic keratoses (AK), squamous cell carcinomas (SCC), basal cell carcinomas (BCC), and corresponding intraindividual controls (IC-AK, IC-SCC, IC-BCC).

Drosha expression levels were normally distributed in all groups. In the BCC group, a highly significant upregulation of Drosha mRNA expression was seen compared to healthy controls ($p < 0.01$) (Fig. 5-3). Compared to intraindividual BCC controls, there were still higher Drosha expression levels, but these differences were not statistically significant ($p > 0.05$). Drosha levels in SCC samples were highly upregulated compared to healthy controls ($p < 0.01$), but not compared to intraindividual controls ($p > 0.05$) (Fig. 5-4). In AK samples, we could not observe any significant differences in Drosha expression compared to either healthy or intraindividual controls ($p > 0.05$).

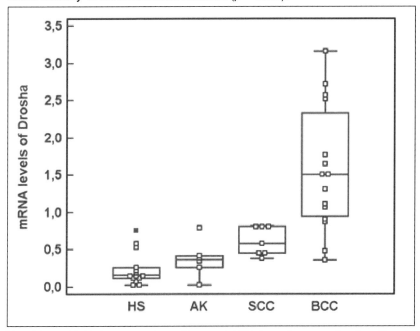

Fig. 5-3:   Multiple comparison Box and Whisker diagram showing Drosha mRNA expression in healthy subjects (HS), actinic keratosis (AK), squamous cell carcinomas (SCC), and basal cell carcinomas (BCC).

No significant difference in Dicer expression levels between intraindividual and healthy controls was observed ($p > 0.05$). However, Drosha expression levels in intraindividual controls were highly upregulated compared to healthy controls (*p* < 0.01). Details of quantitative real-time PCR data are given in Table 5-1.

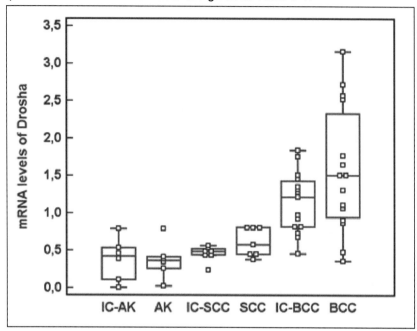

Fig. 5-4:   Multiple comparison Box and Whisker diagram showing Drosha mRNA expression in actinic keratoses (AK), squamous cell carcinomas (SCC), basal cell carcinomas (BCC), and corresponding intraindividual controls (IC-AK, IC-SCC, IC-BCC).

5.4   Discussion

Alterations in the microRNA (miRNA) machinery play important roles in the carcinogenesis of a variety of tumors [8]. Both up- and downregulation of miRNAs have been reported, and changes in the stoichiometry of miRNA machinery components are thought to explain abnormal miRNA profiles in different cancers. However, it is unclear whether the observed up- or downregulation of miRNA expression simply reflects malignant degeneration of the tumor or directly causes tumor initiation and progression. As miRNAs control both oncogenes and tumor suppressors, it remains unclear if and how miRNAs may influence carcinogenesis.

Tab. 5-1: Quantitative real-time RT-PCR data of Dicer (x10) and Drosha (means ± SD) levels investigated in actinic keratoses (AK, n = 6), squamous cell carcinomas (SCC, n = 7), basal cell carcinomas (BCC, n = 15), healthy subjects (HS, n = 14), and corresponding intraindividual (IC) controls of each tumor patient (IC-AK, n = 6; IC-SCC, n = 7; IC-BCC, n = 15), PS = primer sequence used in this study, RPL38 = human R38 ribosomal protein (housekeeping gene). All data are expressed as re-transformed logarithmic values. * = statistically significant difference

Parameter	Drosha HS Control (a)	Drosha IC Control (b)	Drosha AK (c)	Drosha SCC (d)	Drosha BCC (e)
RT-PCR	0.25 ± 0.22 a versus b* a versus d* a versus e*	0.38 ± 0.29 (IC-AK) 0.46 ± 0.11 (IC-BCC) 1.15 ± 0.41 (IC-BCC)	0.37 ± 0.25	0.62 ± 0.2	1.57 ± 0.84
PS Drosha	F 5´-CATGTCACAGAATGTCGTTCCA-3´ ; R 5´-GGGTGAAGCAGCCTCAGATTT-3´				

Parameter	Dicer HS Control (a)	Dicer IC Control (b)	Dicer AK (c)	Dicer SCC (d)	Dicer BCC (e)
RT-PCR	0.089 ± 0.08 a versus e*	0.12 ± 0.15 (IC-AK) 0.05 ± 0.04 (IC-SCC) 0.11 ± 0.09 (IC-BCC) b versus d* b versus e*	0.05 ± 0.04	0.12 ± 0.06	0.06 ± 0.08
PS Dicer	F 5´-TTAACCTTTTGGTGTTTGATGAGTGT-3´ ; R 5´-GGACATGATGGACAATTTTCACA-3´				
PS RPL38	F 5´-TCACTGACAAAGAGAAGGCAGAGA-3´ ; R 5´-TCAGTGTGTCTGGTTCATTTCAGTT-3´				

To investigate the role of miRNAs in the carcinogenesis of epithelial skin cancer, we assessed expression levels of two pivotal enzymes in the miRNA maturation process, Dicer and Drosha. Nevertheless there are also other factors which are necessary for proper pri-miRNA processing and which are subject of current investigation [9]. They include the double-stranded RNA binding protein (dsRBP) known as DiGeorge syndrome critical region 8 (DGCR8) which determines the cleavage sites on the pri-miRNA or the human immunodeficiency virus transactivating response RNA-binding protein (TRBP) which is also a double-stranded RNA binding protein dsRBP necessary loading mature miRNAs into the RISC [10]. However in this exploratory pilot study we investigated the two main enzymes Dicer and Drosha wherefore the other factors could be subject of further studies.

Drosha is an intranuclear RNase III enzyme that cleaves pri-miRNAs into precursor miRNAs (pre-miRNAs). Here, we found a highly significant upregulation of Drosha expression in basal cell carcinomas compared to healthy controls ($p < 0.01$), and interestingly, no significant difference was seen when compared to intraindividual controls. This result supports the hypothesis that patients with BCC may show an alteration in Drosha expression levels not only in the tumor tissue, but also in healthy skin near the tumor border. Taken one step further, we suggest that changes in Drosha expression in the skin of patients with BCC is possible regardless of localization and may be associated with changes in miRNA expression profiles. However, this cannot be assessed based on our data alone, as the intraindividual controls were harvested adjacent to the tumor. Although unlikely, it is possible that patients with BCC show alterations in expression of miRNA machinery components in their skin, which could directly or indirectly promote carcinogenesis depending on the interaction of several factors.

Although cervical squamous cell carcinomas show very different biological behaviors compared to squamous cell carcinomas of the skin, we found interesting similarities in changes of expression of the miRNA machinery [11]. Analogous to our observations in pre-malignant skin lesions (actinic keratoses), Mualidhar et al. also did not observe an increase of Drosha expression in pre-malignant cervical SCC intraepithelial lesions [12]. However, in clinically progressed cervical SCC, Drosha copy-number gain was observed, in agreement with our results showing significantly higher Drosha expression in SCC of the skin compared to healthy controls ($p < 0.01$). Similar to the BCC findings, there was no significant difference when compared to the intraindividual controls, showing that alterations in the miRNA machinery are not solely restricted to the site of the tumor, but also affects the adjacent skin. miRNAs associated with Drosha overexpression are implicated in the carcinogenesis in many other tissues. We therefore hypothesize that miRNAs potentially regulate fundamental processes in neoplastic progression of the skin, as Drosha was significantly overexpressed in both the BCC and SCC groups.

Dicer is a cytosolic enzyme responsible for cutting pre-miRNAs into mature miRNAs and has been recently identified as a critical player in embryonic skin morphogenesis [13]. Furthermore, it has been shown that a disruption of Dicer function leads to disturbance of heterochromatin formation and pericentromeric silencing in different organisms [14,15], which disrupts chromosome segregation and leads to aneuploidies, a characteristic feature of cancer [16]. Upregulation of Dicer has been described for prostate adenocarcinomas and lung carcinomas, while downregulation or lower expression of Dicer was found to be significantly associated with advanced tumor stages of ovarian carcinomas and non-small cell lung cancer [17-20]. However, the potential role of Dicer in skin carcinogenesis has not yet been investigated. In the present pilot study, we showed that Dicer is significantly downregulated in BCC tissue compared to both intraindividual and healthy control samples ($p < 0.05$). In contrast, Dicer was significantly upregulated in SCC compared to intraindividual controls ($p < 0.05$). Chiosea et al. showed that in lung adenocarcinomas, Dicer was downregulated in areas of invasion and in cases of advanced disease. Furthermore, they showed that a fraction of lung adenocarcinomas lose Dicer expression as a result of deletions within the Dicer locus [18]. This may also be the case in the BCC group, which would explain the observed significant downregulation of Dicer expression. Whether genetic variations in the miRNA machinery are associated with the risk of epithelial skin cancer or whether Dicer and Drosha expression levels are concomitantly altered due to epithelial skin cancer remains unclear and needs to be addressed further in future studies.

5.5 Conclusion

To determine whether miRNAs play a crucial role in the carcinogenesis of epithelial skin cancer, we investigated the expression levels of the two most important enzymes of the miRNA machinery, Drosha and Dicer, which were clearly dysregulated when compared to healthy controls. Our results favor the hypothesis that miRNAs are involved in the carcinogenesis of epithelial skin cancer, highlighting the importance of miRNA expression profiles to further investigate the role of miRNA dysregulation in epithelial skin carcinogenesis.

5.6 References

1)   miRNA database mirBase http://microrna.sanger.ac.uk/sequences/

2)   Sand M, Gambichler T, Sand D, et al. MicroRNAs and the skin: tiny players in the body's largest organ. J Dermatol Sci. 2009;53: 169-175.

3)   Yi R, Qin Y, Macara IG, et al. Exportin-5 mediates the nuclear export of pre-microRNAs and short hairpin RNAs. Genes Dev. 2003;17: 3011-3016.

4)   Lee Y, Hur I, Park SY, et al. The role of PACT in the RNA silencing pathway. EMBO J. 2006;25: 522-532.

5)   Song JJ, Liu J, Tolia NH, et al. The crystal structure of the Argonaute2 PAZ domain reveals an RNA binding motif in RNAi effector complexes. Nat Struct Biol. 2003;10: 1026-1032.

6)   Nelson KM, Weiss GJ. MicroRNAs and cancer: past, present, and potential future. Mol Cancer Ther. 2008;7: 3655-3660.

7)   Livak KJ, Schmittgen TD. Analysis of relative gene expression data using real-time quantitative PCR and the 2(-Delta Delta C(T)) Method. Methods 2001;25: 402–408.

8)   Horikawa Y, Wood CG, Yang H, et al. Single nucleotide polymorphisms of microRNA machinery genes modify the risk of renal cell carcinoma. Clin Cancer Res. 2008;14: 7956-7962.

9) Perron MP, Provost P. Protein components of the microRNA pathway and human diseases. Methods Mol Biol. 2009;487:369-85.

10) Daniels SM, Melendez-Peña CE, Scarborough RJ, Daher A, Christensen HS, El Far M, Purcell DF, Lainé S, Gatignol A. Characterization of the TRBP domain required for dicer interaction and function in RNA interference. BMC Mol Biol. 2009; 10:38.

11) Greer BE, Koh WJ, Abu-Rustum N, et al. Cervical cancer. J Natl Compr Canc Netw. 2008;6: 14-36.

12) Muralidhar B, Goldstein LD, Ng G, et al. Global microRNA profiles in cervical squamous cell carcinoma depend on Drosha expression levels. J Pathol. 2007;212: 368-377.

13) Yi R, Pasolli HA, Landthaler M, et al. DGCR8-dependent microRNA biogenesis is essential for skin development. Proc Natl Acad Sci USA. 2009 ;106: 498-502.

14) Kanellopoulou C, Muljo SA, Kung AL, et al. Dicer-deficient mouse embryonic stem cells are defective in differentiation and centromeric silencing. Genes Dev. 2005;19: 489-501.

15) Fukagawa T, Nogami M, Yoshikawa M, et al. Dicer is essential for formation of the heterochromatin structure in vertebrate cells. Nat Cell Biol. 2004;6: 784-791.

16) Kanellopoulou C, Monticelli S. A role for microRNAs in the development of the immune system and in the pathogenesis of cancer. Semin Cancer Biol. 2008;18: 79-88.

17) Chiosea S, Jelezcova E, Chandran U, et al. Up-regulation of dicer, a component of the MicroRNA machinery, in prostate adenocarcinoma. Am J Pathol. 2006; 169: 1812-1820.

18) Chiosea S, Jelezcova E, Chandran U, Luo J, Mantha G, Sobol RW, Dacic S. Overexpression of Dicer in precursor lesions of lung adenocarcinoma. Cancer Res. 2007; 67: 2345-50.

19) Merritt WM, Lin YG, Han LY, Kamat AA, Spannuth WA, Schmandt R, Urbauer D, Pennacchio LA, Cheng JF, Nick AM, Deavers MT, Mourad-Zeidan A, Wang H, Mueller P, Lenburg ME, Gray JW, Mok S, Birrer MJ, Lopez-Berestein G, Coleman RL, Bar-Eli M, Sood AK. Dicer, Drosha, and outcomes in patients with ovarian cancer. N Engl J Med. 2008; 359: 2641-2650.

20) Karube Y, Tanaka H, Osada H, Tomida S, Tatematsu Y, Yanagisawa K, Yatabe Y, Takamizawa J, Miyoshi S, Mitsudomi T, Takahashi T. Reduced expression of Dicer associated with poor prognosis in lung cancer patients. Cancer Sci. 2005; 96: 111-115.

6   Paper 2: Expression levels of the microRNA maturing microprocessor complex component DGCR8 and the RNA-induced silencing complex (RISC) components argonaute-1, argonaute-2, PACT, TARBP1 and TARBP2 in epithelial skin cancer*

6.1   Introduction

microRNAs (miRNAs) are thought to play an important role in the post-transcriptional gene regulation of up to 30% of all human genes [1]. The updated version (V.17) of the miRNA database miRBase currently distinguishes 1424 different human miRNA sequences [2]. miRNAs are capable of regulating gene expression both by promoting mRNA degradation and by inhibiting mRNA translation [3]. The maturation of miRNAs occurs in the nucleus and the cytoplasm. The process begins in the nucleus, where the intranuclear enzyme Drosha, an RNase III endonuclease, cleaves pri-miRNAs (consisting of a hairpin stem, a terminal loop, and 5` and 3` single-stranded RNA extensions) to pre-miRNAs (60-70 nucleotide stem-loop structures). In addition to Drosha, the DiGeorge syndrome critical region gene 8 (DGCR8 or Pasha), which is the product of a gene deleted in DiGeorge syndrome, is also part of the miRNA maturing microprocessor complex and has been shown to be essential for miRNA maturation [4]. While Drosha functions as the catalytic subunit of the microprocessor complex, DGCR8 stabilizes Drosha through protein-protein interactions and is responsible for recognition of the RNA substrate [5,6]. The resulting pre-miRNAs are transported into the cytoplasm by Exportin 5 [7]. Here, Dicer, another RNase III enzyme, cleaves the pre-miNAs into mature miRNAs [8]. The intracellular effects of miRNAs are achieved by the RNA-induced silencing complex (RISC), a 200- to 500-kDa multiprotein effector complex with endonuclease activity, which integrates mature miRNA strands. The incorporated miRNA guides the RISC to its specific mRNA

---

* Co-authors: Marina Skrygan Ph.D., Christoph Arenz Ph.D., Dimitrios Georgas M.D., Thilo Gambichler M.D., Daniel Sand M.D., Peter Altmeyer M.D., Falk G. Bechara M.D.

target through base-pair complementation. Once the miRNA has annealed to the target mRNA (near-perfect hybridization), the RISC disrupts translation by cleaving the target mRNA [9]. Weaker hybridization leads to translational repression or degradation of the mRNA [10]. The RISC is the central element of the RNA silencing pathway and consists of several different proteins that comprise a multiprotein complex. The best-characterized RISC proteins include the methyltransferase TARBP1 (TAR [HIV-1] RNA binding protein), the RISC-loading complex subunit TARBP2 (TAR [HIV-1] RNA binding protein), the RISC core components argonaute-1 (AGO1, eukaryotic translation initiation factor 2C.1, EIF2C1) and argonaute-2 (AGO2, eukaryotic translation initiation factor 2C.2, EIF2C2) and the dsRNA-binding protein PACT.

TARBPs are double-stranded RNA binding proteins (dsRBP) that load short RNAs into the RISC [10] and enhance the stability of Dicer-substrate complexes [11]. The argonaute proteins function as the slicer enzymes that cleave mRNA targets after miRNA-mediated complementation, which leads to message degradation [12]. The dsRNA-binding protein PACT binds and activates the interferon-induced protein kinase PKR, which plays a major role in the cellular antiviral defense in mammals and is a component of the human RISC [8,13].

The dysregulated expression of two important miRNA machinery enzymes, Drosha and Dicer, has recently been shown in epithelial skin tumors. As a result, it was hypothesized that the miRNA pathway is involved in the carcinogenesis of epithelial skin cancer, as has been proposed in a variety of other malignancies of the skin and other tissues [14-16]. Because the intracellular role of miRNAs is closely related to RISC function, we initiated the present pilot study to survey the expression levels of the RISC and the microprocessor core components and identify the possible role of miRNAs in epithelial skin cancer and its premalignant stage.

6.2   Materials and Methods

This study was approved by the Ethical Review Board of the Ruhr-University Bochum, Germany (registration number: 3265-08,

ClinicalTrials.gov Identifier: NCT01345760). Twenty-eight patients (10 females, 18 males; median age: 69.9 years) with epithelial skin cancer (15 basal cell carcinomas (BCC), 7 squamous cell carcinomas (SCC)) or premalignant skin lesions (6 actinic keratoses (AK)), all of whom signed an informed consent, were enrolled in the present study. During removal of the skin tumors, which was performed under local anesthesia, a 3-mm punch biopsy was taken from the center of the tumor. A biopsy of healthy skin adjacent to the tumor served as an intraindividual control. A group of 16 healthy subjects (11 females, 5 males; median age: 61.9 years) served as an interindividual control group. After all of the specimens were collected, total cellular RNA was isolated from skin tissue samples with an RNeasy Lipid Tissue Kit (Qiagen, Chatsworth, CA, USA) following the manufacturer's protocol. A $Power$SYBR$^{®}$ Green PCR Master Mix and StepOne™ Real-Time PCR System (Applied Biosystems, Foster City, CA, USA) were used for quantitative analysis with real-time RT-PCR. The necessary PCR primers for DGCR8, argonaute-1, argonaute-2, PACT, TARBP1, TARBP2 and the RPL38 housekeeping gene were designed with the help of Primer Express software (PE Applied Biosystems, Foster City, CA, USA) and produced by the custom oligonucleotide synthesis service TIB Molbiol (Berlin, Germany). The expression data were analyzed using the comparative ΔC_t method described by Livak and Schmittgen [17]. We used the mean expression of the housekeeping gene RPL38 as a control to normalize the variability in the expression levels. The ΔC_t values (logarithms) were re-transformed, and the expression data were multiplied by a factor of 10 to better illustrate mRNA quantities.

Statistical analyses

Data analysis was performed using Med-Calc software version 11.5.1.0 (Mariakerke, Belgium). The null hypothesis was based on the assump tion that there was no difference between the DGCR8, argonaute-1, argonaute-2, PACT, TARBP1 and TARBP2 expression levels in the BCC, SCC and AK specimens compared to healthy interindividual and intraindividual controls. After analysis of the data by the Kolmogorov-Smirnov test revealed a normal distribution, tumor groups were compared with the non-lesional, intraindividual control using two-sided, paired t-tests. To compare tumor groups with healthy interindividual controls, the data were analyzed using two-sided, unpaired t-tests if they fit a normal distribution. In cases of non-normal distributions (such as for argonaute 2 in the BCC group), the data were analyzed using the Mann-Whitney test for independent samples (interindividual control) and the Wilcoxon test for dependent samples (intraindividual control). All of the results were expressed as the mean ± standard deviation (SD), with statistical significance set at 5% (two-sided).

6.3   Results

The DGCR8 expression levels in both the SCC and BCC samples were significantly higher than the intraindividual control samples that did not have lesions ($p<0.05$) (Fig 6-1a). The DGCR8 expression levels were also significantly higher in the BCC samples than in the healthy interindividual control samples ($p<0.05$). The DGCR8 levels in the AK group did not significantly differ from those in the non-lesional intraindividual controls ($p>0.05$). The DGCR8 levels were significantly higher in the BCC interindividual controls than in the non-lesional intraindividual controls ($p<0.05$).

The PACT and argonaute-1 expression levels were significantly higher in the AK, SCC and BCC groups than in the healthy controls ($p<0.05$) (Fig 6-1b and 6-1c). The PACT, argonaute-1 and TARBP2 expression levels in the BCC, SCC and AK groups were not significantly different compared to the non-lesional intraindividual controls ($p>0.05$).

The argonaute-2 expression levels in the SCC samples were significantly higher than the non-lesional intraindividual controls ($p<0.05$) (Fig 6-1d). Compared to the healthy control group, the AK, SCC and BCC groups had significantly higher argonaute-2 expression levels ($p<0.05$). The argonaute-2 levels in the BCC and AK groups were not significantly different compared to the non-lesional intraindividual controls ($p>0.05$). The PACT, argonaute-1 and argonaute-2 expression levels were significantly higher in the AK, SCC and BCC interindividual controls than in the non-lesional intraindividual controls ($p<0.05$).

The TARBP1 expression levels in the AK samples were significantly higher than in the non-lesional intraindividual controls ($p<0.05$) (Fig 6-1e). The TARBP1 expression levels in the BCC and SCC groups were not significantly different compared to the non-lesional intraindividual controls ($p>0.05$). The TARBP2 expression levels in the BCC, SCC and AK groups were not significantly different compared to the non-lesional intraindividual controls ($p>0.05$) or healthy controls ($p>0.05$) (Fig 6-1f). However, the TARBP2 expression levels were significantly higher in the BCC interindividual controls compared to the non-lesional intraindividual controls ($p<0.05$). Details of the quantitative real-time PCR data are given in Table 6-1.

6.4   Discussion

miRNA pathways regulate gene expression by inducing degradation and/or translational repression of target mRNAs. Perturbations in the miRNA machinery have been linked to carcinogenesis in a variety of different tumors [18]. However, there has been little research conducted on the role of miRNAs in epithelial skin cancer. In a recent pilot study, the intranuclear enzyme Drosha, which is a major component of the miRNA maturing microprocessor complex, was upregulated in epithelial skin cancer. This was true for both basal cell and squamous cell carcinoma [14]. Drosha upregulation has also been found in clinically aggressive cervical SCC [19]. Based on these initial findings, this study was performed to further investigate possible perturbations of other well-defined components of the miRNA machinery in epithelial skin cancer.

In the present study, we showed that DGCR8, an essential Drosha cofactor and an essential part of the miRNA maturing microprocessor complex, has significantly higher expression in SCC and BCC compared to non-lesional skin samples ($p<0.05$) and in BCC compared to healthy controls. DGCR8 works closely with Drosha in a 650-kDa microprocessor complex, which is essential for miRNA maturation [20]. RISC is the effector complex of the miRNA pathway. PACT, an essential component of the RISC, showed significantly increased expression levels in all investigated groups (AK, SCC, BCC) compared to healthy controls. In addition to its essential function in the RISC, PACT is a stimulus inducing dsRNA-dependent protein kinase (PKR) that mediates apoptosis [21]. PKR has been associated with anti-viral (antitumor) and apoptotic responses and has been shown to be increased after ultraviolet (UV) stress, an important etiologic factor in epithelial skin carcinogenesis [22].

The highly conserved argonaute proteins, which were investigated in the present study, are also a pivotal part of the RISC, the effector complex of the miRNA pathway. The argonautes are the heart of the effector RISC complex and function as slicer enzymes, cleaving mRNA targets. The elevated expression of argonaute-2 has been described for head and neck SCC [23,24]. Our data show that argonaute-2 is also significantly overexpressed in skin SCC, as was previously shown for Dicer ($p<0.05$), which is also overexpressed in skin SCC [14]. This was as expected because Dicer and argonaute-2 are both part of the RISC and overexpression of only one RISC component would have been unlikely. Another important component of the RISC that showed increased expression in AK and SCC is TARBP1, a 185-kDa protein product of a gene located on chromosome 1. TARBP1 belongs to the RNA methyltransferase trmH family and is responsible for Dicer stability and for the proper assembly of RISC; it facilitates the loading of miRNAs onto the RISC. TARBP2 is the product of a gene located on chromosome 12 and is a 39-kDa protein component of the RISC complex. In the present study, expression of TARBP2 was not significantly different for the cancer groups compared to the controls. One possible explanation is that some enzymes and cofactors that are involved in miRNA processing pathways, such as TARBP2, may be targets of genetic disruption. TARBP2 mutations recently were described in human cancers and could result in impaired microRNA processing and Dicer function without affecting the actual quantity of expression [25].

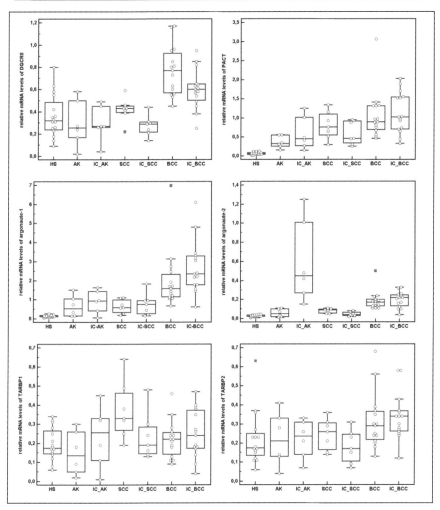

Fig. 6-1: Multiple comparison Box-and-Whisker plot showing DGCR8 (a), PACT (b), argonaute-1 (c), argonaute- 2 (d), TARBP1 (e), and TARBP2 (f) mRNA expression relative to RPL38 mRNA expression in healthy subjects (HS) and patients with actinic keratoses (AK), squamous cell carcinomas (SCC), and basal cell carcinomas (BCC) as well as their corresponding intraindividual controls (IC-AK, IC-SCC, IC-BCC).

Tab. 6-1: Quantitative real-time RT-PCR data of DGCR8, argonaute-1, argonaute-2, PACT, TARBP1 and TARBP2 (mean ± SD) expression levels investigated in actinic keratosis (AK, n = 6), squamous cell carcinoma (SCC, n = 7), basal cell carcinoma (BCC, n = 15), healthy subjects (HS, n = 16) and the corresponding intraindividual (IC) controls for each tumor patient (IC-AK, n = 6; IC-SCC, n = 7; IC-BCC, n = 15) relative to RPL38 expression; PS = primer sequence used in this study, RPL38 = human ribosomal protein R38 (housekeeping gene). All data are re-transformed ΔCt values (logarithms). * = statistically significant difference

Parameter	DGCR8 HS Control (a)	DGCR8 IC Control (b)	DGCR8 AK (c)	DGCR8 SCC (d)	DGCR8 BCC (e)
RT-PCR	0.36 ± 0.19	0.3 ± 0.16 (IC-AK)	0.3 ± 0.21	0.42 ± 0.11	0.77 ± 0.22
		0.28 ± 0.09 (IC-SCC)			
		0.6 ± 0.18 (IC-BCC)			
	a versus b (IC-BCC) * a versus e*	b versus d* b versus e*			
PS DGCR8	F-5´-gcaagatgcacccacaaaga-3´; R-5´-ttgaggacacgctgcatgtac-3´				

Parameter	AGO1 HS Control (a)	AGO1 IC Control (b)	AGO1 AK (c)	AGO1 SCC (d)	AGO1 BCC (e)
RT-PCR	0.14 ± 0.05	0.9 ± 0.6 (IC-AK) 0.75 ± 0.57 (IC-SCC) 2.7 ± 1.4 (IC-BCC)	0.65 ± 0.55	0.64 ± 0.36	2.0 ± 1.53
	a versus b (IC-AK)* a versus b (IC-SCC)* a versus b (IC-BCC)* a versus c* a versus d* a versus e*				
PS AGO1	F-5´-gatccctgttcccttggagtct-3´; R-5´- tcaggcggtgagaagaagga-3´				

Tab. 6-1: (Continued)

Parameter	AGO2 HS Control (a)	AGO2 IC Control (b)	AGO2 AK (c)	AGO2 SCC (d)	AGO2 BCC (e)
RT-PCR	0.03 ± 0.01	0.07 ± 0.05 (IC-AK) 0.05 ± 0.02 (IC-SCC) 0.2 ± 0.08 (IC-BCC)	0.06 ± 0.04	0.08 ± 0.02	0.39 ± 0.8
	a versus b (IC-AK)* a versus b (IC-SCC)* a versus b (IC-BCC)* a versus c* a versus d* a versus e*	b versus d*			
PS AGO2	F-5´-tcatggtcaaagatgagatgacaga-3´; R-5´-tttattcctgcccccgtaga-3´				

Parameter	PACT HS Control (a)	PACT IC Control (b)	PACT AK (c)	PACT SCC(d)	PACT BCC (e)
RT-PCR	0.07 ± 0.04	0.6 ± 0.44 (IC-AK) 0.6 ± 0.3 (IC-SCC) 1.13 ± 0.53 (IC-BCC)	0.36 ± 0.16	0.81 ± 0.36	1.06 ± 0.63
	a versus b (IC-AK)* a versus b (IC-SCC)* a versus b (IC-BCC)* a versus c* a versus d* a versus e*				
PS PACT	F- 5´-tgcagttcctgaccccttaatg-3´; R-5´-agccaattcctgtaatgaaccaa-3´				

Tab. 6-1: (Continued)

Parameter	TARBP1 HS Control (a)	TARBP1 IC Control (b)	TARBP1 AK (c)	TARBP1 SCC (d)	TARBP1 BCC (e)
RT-PCR	0.2 ± 0.08 a versus d*	0.24 ± 0.16 (IC-AK) 0.23 ± 0.12 (IC-SCC) 0.25 ± 0.13 (IC-BCC) b versus c*	0.15 ± 0.11	0.37 ± 0.15	0.22 ± 0.1
PS TARBP1	F 5´-cattaatggatgcgctttcaga-3´; R 5´-tgtaatttcagtcccaatggagaac-3´				

Parameter	TARBP2 HS Control (a)	TARBP2 IC Control (b)	TARBP2 AK (c)	TARBP2 SCC (d)	TARBP2 BCC (e)
RT-PCR	0.22 ± 0.14 a versus b (IC-BCC)*	0.22 ± 0.1 (IC-AK) 0.18 ± 0.09 (IC-SCC) 0.34 ± 0.12 (IC-BCC)	0.22 ± 0.14	0.25 ± 0.08	0.32 ± 0.15
PS TARBP2	F 5´-ggttgccggagtacacagtga-3´; R 5´-tgccactcccaatctcaatg-3´				
PS RPL 38	F 5´-tcactgacaaagagaaggcagaga-3´ ; R 5´-tcagtgtgtctggttcatttcagtt-3´				

The findings of our study show that the expression of important miRNA machinery components, such as the microprocessor complex and RISC components, is disturbed in epithelial skin cancer, as was previously shown for Dicer and Drosha. However, based on our data, it is not possible to resolve whether these findings can be regarded as an epiphenomenon or have a causative effect on the pathogenesis of epithelial skin cancer. Given that the argonaute-1, argonaute-2 and PACT levels are significantly elevated in the unaffected tissues of AK, SCC and BCC patients, as are the DGCR8 and TARBP2 levels in the unaffected tissues of BCC patients, one may speculate that the increased mRNA expression is a non-sufficient condition (or a causative factor) for pathogenesis rather than a consequence of transformation. Nevertheless, this study has shown that essential miRNA pathway components, such as the RISC and the microprocessor complexes, are disrupted in epithelial skin cancer, and their possible role in carcinogenesis should be further investigated.

6.5   Conclusion

This study was performed to determine whether the mature miRNA microprocessor complex component DGCR8 and the RISC components argonaute-1, argonaute-2, PACT, TARBP1 and TARBP2 play a role in the carcinogenesis of epithelial skin cancer. Combined, the findings indicate that the miRNA pathway is dysregulated in epithelial skin cancer carcinogenesis and should be further investigated.

6.6   References

1)   Lewis BP, Burge CB, Bartel DP. Conserved seed pairing, often flanked by adenosines, indicates that thousands of human genes are microRNA targets. Cell 2005;120:15-20.

2)   http://www.mirbase.org/ (accessed August 2011)

3)   Bartel DP. MicroRNAs: genomics, biogenesis, mechanism, and function. Cell 2004;116:281-297.

4)   Gregory RI, Yan KP, Amuthan G, et al. The Microprocessor complex mediates the genesis of microRNAs. Nature 2004;432: 235-240.

5)   Han J, Pedersen JS, Kwon SC, et al. Posttranscriptional crossregulation between Drosha and DGCR8. Cell 2009;136:75-84.

6) Wang Y, Medvid R, Melton C, Jaenisch R, Blelloch R. DGCR8 is essential for microRNA biogenesis and silencing of embryonic stem cell self-renewal. Nat Genet 2007;39:380-385.

7) Yi R, Qin Y, Macara IG, et al. Exportin-5 mediates the nuclear export of pre-microRNAs and short hairpin RNAs. Genes Dev 2003;17:3011-3016.

8) Lee Y, Hur I, Park SY, Kim YK, Suh MR, Kim VN. The role of PACT in the RNA silencing pathway. EMBO J 2006;25:522-532.

9) Dalmay T. MicroRNAs and cancer. J Intern Med 2008;263:366-375.

10) Daniels SM, Melendez-Peña CE, Scarborough RJ, et al. Characterization of the TRBP domain required for dicer interaction and function in RNA interference. BMC Mol Biol 2009;10:38.

11) Chakravarthy S, Sternberg SH, Kellenberger CA, Doudna JA. Substrate-specific kinetics of Dicer-catalyzed RNA processing. J Mol Biol. 2010;404:392-402.

12) Faehnle CR, Joshua-Tor L. Argonautes confront new small RNAs. Curr Opin Chem Biol 2007;11:569-577.

13) Peters GA, Seachrist DD, Keri RA, Sen GC. The double-stranded RNA-binding protein, PACT, is required for postnatal anterior pituitary proliferation. Proc Natl Acad Sci USA 2009;106:10696-11701.

14) Sand M, Gambichler T, Skrygan M, Sand D, Altmeyer P, Bechara FG. Expression levels of microRNA processing enzymes Drosha and Dicer in epithelial skin cancer. Cancer Investigation 2010;28:649-653.

15) Sand M, Gambichler T, Sand D, Altmeyer P, Stuecker M, Bechara FG. Immunhistochemical expression patterns of the microRNA processing enzyme Dicer in cutaneous malignant melanoma, benign and dysplastic melanocytic naevi. Eur J Dermatol 2011;21:18-21.

16) Sand M, Gambichler T, Sand D, Skrygan M, Altmeyer P, Bechara FG. MicroRNAs and the skin: Tiny players in the body's largest organ. J Dermatol Sci 2009;53:169-175.

17) Livak KJ, Schmittgen TD. Analysis of relative gene expression data using real-time quantitative PCR and the 2(-Delta Delta C(T)) Method. Methods 2001;25:402–408.

18) Gartel AL, Kandel ES. RNA interference in cancer. Biomol Eng 2006;23:17-34.

19) Muralidhar B, Goldstein LD, Ng G, et al. Global microRNA profiles in cervical squamous cell carcinoma depend on Drosha expression levels. J Pathol 2007;212:368-377.

20) Han J, Lee Y, Yeom KH, Kim YK, Jin H, Kim VN. The Drosha-DGCR8 complex in primary microRNA processing. Genes Dev 2004;18:3016-3027.

21) Ito T, Yang M, May S. RAX, a cellular activator for double-stranded RNA dependent protein kinase during stress signaling. J Biol Chem 1999;274:15427–15432.

22) Zykova TA, Zhu F, Zhang Y, Bode AM, Dong Z. Involvement of ERKs, RSK2 and PKR in UVA-induced signal transduction toward phosphorylation of eIF2alpha (Ser(51)). Carcinogenesis 2007;28:1543-1551.

23) Li L, Yu C, Gao H, Li Y. Argonaute proteins: potential biomarkers for human colon cancer. BMC Cancer 2010;10:38.

24) Chang SS, Smith I, Glazer C, Hennessey P, Califano JA. EIF2C is overexpressed and amplified in head and neck squamous cell carcinoma. ORL J Otorhinolaryngol Relat Spec 2010;72:337-343.

25) Melo SA, Ropero S, Moutinho C, et al. A TARBP2 mutation in human cancer impairs microRNA processing and DICER1 function. Nat Genet 2009;41:365-370.

7 Paper 3: Expression of microRNAs in basal cell carcinoma*

7.1 Introduction

Basal cell carcinoma (BCC) of the skin is the most common cancer in humans. Although first described by Krompecher in 1900, the molecular pathogenesis of BCC has yet to be completely understood [1]. A variety of different tumor-promoting signaling cascades, including the Hedgehog (HH) and the MAPK/ERK pathways, have been reported to play a role in BCC development [2].

MicroRNAs (miRNAs) are a relatively new class of short RNAs that are involved in post-transcriptional gene regulation, but they have not been extensively studied with respect to the molecular pathogenesis of BCC. Because it is estimated that 30 – 60 % of all human genes are controlled by miRNAs, a potential role for miRNAs in the molecular pathogenesis of BCC deserves investigation. As a class, miRNAs have been implicated in a variety of physiological and pathophysiological processes of the skin and other tissues of the human body [3]. Recently, the miRNA maturing enzymes Drosha and Dicer as well as pivotal parts of the miRNA microprocessor complex and the miRNA effector RNA-induced silencing complex (RISC) were reported to be dysregulated in epithelial skin tumors, including BCC [4,5]. Based on these preliminary reports of alterations in the miRNA machinery, we initiated a microarray-based miRNA profiling study to identify specific miRNA candidates that are differentially expressed in BCC.

7.2 Materials and Methods

The present study was approved by the Ethical Review Board of the Ruhr-University Bochum, Germany (registration number: 3265-08, ClinicalTrials.gov Identifier: NCT01498250) and originated from a dermatologic surgery section at an academic university hospital. This

---

* Co-authors: Marina Skrygan Ph.D., Daniel Sand M.D., Dimitrios Georgas M.D., Stephan Hahn M.D., Thilo Gambichler M.D., Peter Altmeyer M.D., Falk G. Bechara M.D.

study was designed and performed within the framework of the declaration of Helsinki, and all study subjects signed informed consent.

7.2.1   Subjects

Seven patients (3 females, 4 males; median age: 69.9 years) with basal cell carcinoma were enrolled in this study (Tab. 7-1). Concurrent to excising the BCCs with cold steel under local anesthesia, 4-mm punch biopsies were taken from the center of the tumor and from adjacent non-lesional epithelial skin (NLES, control); these samples were immediately placed in RNAlater (Qiagen, Hilden, Germany) and stored at -80 °C.

7.2.2   RNA isolation

Total RNA, including miRNAs, was isolated with the miRNeasy Mini Kit (Qiagen, Hilden, Germany) according to the manufacturer's protocol. RNA concentration, purity and RNA integrity number (RIN) were determined on a NanoDrop ND-1000 spectrophotometer (Peqlab, Erlangen, Germany), an Agilent 2100 Bioanalyzer and RNA 6000 NanoLabChip Kits (both Agilent Technologies, Santa Clara, USA). The inclusion criteria required a minimum RIN $\geq$ 6.0 for the sample to be acceptable for microarray analysis.

7.2.3   Preparation of labeled miRNA, microarray hybridization and scanning

Total RNA samples were spiked using the MicroRNA Spike-In Kit (Agilent Technologies, Santa Clara, USA) to assess the labeling and hybridization efficiencies. After the spiked total RNA was treated with alkaline calf intestine phosphatase (CIP), a labeling reaction was initiated with 100 ng total RNA per sample. T4 RNA ligase, which incorporates cyanine 3-cytidine biphosphate (miRNA Complete Labeling and Hyb Kit, Agilent Technologies, Santa Clara, USA), was used to label the dephosphorylated RNA.

Tab. 7-1: Details of BCC and control specimen.
mm=millimeters, BCC= basal cell carcinoma, RIN= RNA integrity number. n.a.= not applicable

Sample ID	Sex	Age	Localisation	Histology	Invasion depth	RNA conc. (ng/µl)	A260/280 ratio	RIN
1_BCC	w	96	scalp	solid BCC	6.7 mm	1258.30	2.08	7.5
1_control	w	96	scalp	non-lesional epithelial skin	n.a.	157.66	2.06	8.2
2_BCC	m	65	cheek	solid BCC	4.6 mm	497.06	2.04	7.1
2_control	m	65	cheek	non-lesional epithelial skin	n.a.	114.77	2.06	7.6
3_BCC	w	62	forearm	solid BCC	6.4 mm	210.74	2.07	8.2
3_control	w	62	forearm	non-lesional epithelial skin	n.a.	35.19	2.10	6.0
4_BCC	m	81	popliteal	solid BCC	19.6 mm	3595.21	1.78	8.9
4_control	m	81	popliteal	non-lesional epithelial skin	n.a.	343.37	2.05	8.1
5_BCC	w	38	scalp	multicentric	3.2 mm	310.64	2.07	8.9
5_control	w	38	scalp	non-lesional epithelial skin	n.a.	51.11	1.92	8.2
6_BCC	m	61	thorax	solid BCC	3.1 mm	1617.81	2.10	6.4
6_control	m	61	thorax	non-lesional epithelial skin	n.a.	81.47	2.09	7.1
7_BCC	m	86	preauricular	solid BCC	2.7 mm	140.47	2.02	6.0
7_control	m	86	preauricular	non-lesional epithelial skin	n.a.	116.26	2.10	6.4

Cyanine-3-labeled miRNA samples were subsequently prepared for one-color hybridization (Complete miRNA Labeling and Hyb Kit, Agilent Technologies, Santa Clara, USA). The labeled miRNA samples were hybridized to human miRNA microarrays (Release 16.0, 8x60K format) (Agilent Technologies, Santa Clara, USA) at 55°C for 20 hrs. After washing the microarray slides with increasing stringency (Gene Expression Wash Buffers, Agilent Technologies, Santa Clara), they were dried with acetonitrile (Sigma-Aldrich, St. Louis, USA). Fluorescent signal intensities were detected on an Agilent DNA Microarray Scanner (Agilent Technologies, Santa Clara, USA) with the Scan Control A.8.4.1 Software (Agilent Technologies, Santa Clara, USA) and extracted from the images using the Feature Extraction 10.7.3.1 Software (Agilent Technologies, Santa Clara, USA). All of the steps described were performed according to the manufacturer´s instructions.

7.2.4   *TaqMan quantitative real-time reverse transcription polymerase chain reaction (qRT-PCR)*

To validate the microarray data, the expression of seven miRNAs (5 up-regulated and 2 down-regulated) and the reference gene U6 snRNA was analyzed using TaqMan qRT-PCR with inventoried made-to-order TaqMan microRNA assays (Applied Biosystems, Darmstadt, Germany).

The qRT-PCR analysis was performed in technical replicates according to the manufacturer's instructions using the TaqMan Universal MasterMix II no UNG (Applied Biosystems, Darmstadt, Germany) in a final reaction volume of 10 µl. The reaction mix was transferred into 384-well plates that were run on an AB7900HT instrument (Applied Biosystems, Darmstadt, Germany). The software SDS 2.4 (Applied Biosystems, Darmstadt, Germany) was utilized for instrument control, data acquisition and raw data analysis. The plates were run in relative quantification ($\Delta\Delta C_t$) mode with triplicate measurements and the following temperature profile: 50°C / 2:00 min – 95°C / 10:00 min – 40 cycles x [95°C / 0:15 min – 60°C / 1:00 min]. To calculate the relative expression levels of the target miRNAs, the $\Delta\Delta C_t$ method was applied as previously described by Zhang et al [6]. The fold changes of the selected miRNAs were transformed to $\log_2$ values ($\log_2$ (qRT-PCR) and $\log_2$

(microarray)) to correlate the qRT-PCR and microarray results. Pearson´s correlation coefficient r and a two-sample paired t-test (significance level set at p < 0.05) were calculated.

7.2.5   Bioinformatic data analyses

The data from this study have been deposited in NCBI's Gene Expression Omnibus (GEO) and are accessible through GEO Series accession number GSE34535 (Internet address: http://www.ncbi.nlm.nih. gov/geo/query/acc.cgi?acc=GSE34535) [7]. For quality control, statistical analysis, miRNA annotation and visualization purposes, we used Feature Extraction 10.7.3.1 and GeneSpring GX 11.5.1 (both Agilent Technologies, Santa Clara, USA). Quantile normalization was applied to the data set to obtain an equal distribution of probe signal intensities. Pearson's correlation coefficient (r) was calculated for each sample within the two groups and for all pair-wise comparisons. Cluster analysis was performed using the unweighted pair-group method with arithmetic mean (UPGMA) based on Euclidean distance with hierarchical clustering applied to the normalized data [8,9]. The normalized and $\log_2$ transformed data were averaged across the specimen, and a pair-wise comparison was performed between non-lesional epithelial skin (used as the reference group) and BCC.

7.2.6   Statistical analyses

We performed a paired t-test after adjusting the original p-value by applying the algorithm devised by Benjamini and Hochberg [10]. Fold changes were calculated to identify differential expression between the BCC and control groups. The normalized signal values were transformed from the $\log_2$ to the linear scale. To identify miRNAs differentially expressed in BCC versus control, statistical significance and robust detection were evaluated. Statistical significance was defined by a p value dependent on whether a stringent or a non-stringent filtering approach was applied. In the stringent filtering approach, a probe was classified as induced if the corrected p-value was ≤ 0.05 with a fold change ≥ 2.0 and as repressed if the corrected p-value was ≤ 0.05 with a fold change ≥ - 2.0. In the non-stringent filtering approach, a probe was

classified as induced if the non-adjusted p-value was ≤ 0.01 and 0.05
with a fold change ≥ 2.0 and repressed if the non-adjusted p-value was ≤
0.01 and 0.05 with a fold change ≥ - 2.0.

7.2.7   Data mining analysis

For the data mining analysis of differentially expressed miRNAs found by
the stringent filtering approach, we utilized the following databases and
miRNA target prediction sites: the human miRNA-associated disease
database HMDD (http://cmbi.bjmu.edu.cn/hmdd), the miRNA database
for miRNA functional annotations miRDB (http://mirdb.org/miRDB), the
Target Scan Human for prediction of miRNA targets (http://www.
targetscan.org/), the Mir2Disease database (http://www.mir2disease.
org/) [11], the miRò miRNA knowledge base (http://ferrolab.dmi.unict.
it/miro), PubMed (http://www.ncbi.nlm.nih.gov/pubmed/) and the miRNA
database miRBase (http://www.mirbase.org).

7.3   Results

7.3.1   Quality control

Feature extraction software 10.7.3.1 (Agilent Technologies, Santa Clara,
USA) generated quality control (QC) reports for each array. All of the
quality criteria for successful microarray analysis, as predefined by the
manufacturer, were fulfilled for each array. Visual inspection of the
corner spots in the QC reports confirmed correct automatic corner
finding and grid placing for all arrays.

7.3.2   Differential miRNA expression based on microarray data

After applying a stringent filtering approach that compared BCC with
NLES (adjusted p value ≤ 0.05, fold change ≥ 2.0), we identified sixteen
up-regulated and ten down-regulated miRNAs. The upregulated miRNAs
were as follows: hsa-miR-17, miR-18a, hsa-miR-18b, hsa-miR-19b, hsa-
miR-19b-1*, hsa-miR-93, hsa-miR-106b, hsa-miR-125a-5p, hsa-miR-
130a, hsa-miR-181c, hsa-miR-181c*, hsa-miR-181d, hsa-miR-182, hsa-
miR-455-3p, hsa-miR-455-5p and hsa-miR-542-5p. The down-regulated
miRNAs were as follows: hsa-miR-29c, hsa-miR-29c*, hsa-miR-139-5p,

hsa-miR-140-3p, hsa-miR-145, hsa-miR-378, hsa-miR-572, hsa-miR-638, hsa-miR-2861 and hsa-miR-3196. Tab. 7-2 and 7-3 contain additional details.

7.3.3   Correlation analysis

All samples in this study had a medium-to-high correlation when they were compared between and within each group. Pearson´s correlation coefficient r ranged from 0.939 to 0.977 with an average of 0.952 for samples within the BCC group and from 0.852 to 0.978 with an average of 0.929 for samples within the control group. When comparing the BCC group with the control group, r ranged from 0.834 to 0.963 with an average of 0.914. The results of the correlation analyses are summarized in Tab. 7-4 and Fig. 7-1.

Tab. 7-2:   Total number of differentially expressed miRNAs. First column adjusted p value (adj.-p), second and third column non-adjusted p value (p), basal cell carcinoma (BCC)

Comparison	adj.-p $\leq$ 0.05 $|FC| \geq 2.0$		p $\leq$ 0.01 $|FC| \geq 2.0$		p $\leq$ 0.05 $|FC| \geq 2.0$	
	Up	Down	Up	Down	Up	Down
BCC vs. control	16	10	22	21	51	40

7.3.4   Cluster analysis

Cluster analysis revealed a high degree of similarity among all samples in this study. Nevertheless, heat map analysis and hierarchical clustering placed BBC samples 2_BCC, 3_BCC, 4_BCC, 5_BCC, 6_BCC and 7_BCC closest together. Samples 2_control, 3_control and 6_control were the most dissimilar compared with the other eleven samples in this study. Overall, we observed a heterogeneous miRNA expression profile (Fig. 7-2).

7.3.5 TaqMan qRT-PCR validation

To validate the microarray data acquired using TaqMan qRT-PCR, the reference gene U6 snRNA and the following seven differentially expressed miRNAs were evaluated: hsa-miR-17, hsa-miR-181c, hsa-miR-455-3p, hsa-miR-455-5p and hsa-miR-182 (all up-regulated) and hsa-miR-378 and hsa-miR-139-5p (both down-regulated). The differential expression of the target miRNAs between BCC and control is summarized in Fig. 7-3. Pearson´s correlation coefficient r and the p value based on a two-sample paired t-test were calculated using the $\log_2$ fold changes from the qRT-PCR and microarray results. The qRT-PCR and microarray results were highly correlated, with Pearson´s correlation coefficient r= 0.95 and p= 0.251 showing no significant difference (p > 0.05) between the two assays (Fig. 7-4).

7.3.6 Data mining results

A PubMed search identified no previous BCC miRNA profiling studies. We describe and discuss the findings of our mining data analysis within the discussion section.

7.4 Discussion

Despite the fact that BCC is the most common type of cancer in humans, there is little information about its molecular pathogenesis. Defects in the Hedgehog (HH) and the mitogen activated protein kinase (MAPK/ERK) signaling pathways have been found to play a carcinogenic role in the molecular pathogenesis of BCC [12].

Tab. 7-3: Comparison of BCC vs. control, significantly up- and down-regulated miRNAs sorted by their FC= fold change, BCC= basal cell carcinoma

Comparison	adj.-p ≤ 0.05 |FC| ≥ 2.0						
BCC vs. control	Up				Down			
	16				10			
BCC vs. control (miRNA detail)	miRNA	Fold change	p-value		miRNA	Fold change	p-value	
	hsa-miR-455-5p	+208,65079	0,0041327		hsa-miR-139-5p	-62,62671	0,0041327	
	hsa-miR-181c	+152,5843	0,00479409		hsa-miR-378	-33,490833	0,04645431	
	hsa-miR-181d	+84,06773	0,005365		hsa-miR-29c*	-19,222433	0,0412766	
	hsa-miR-182	+70,646385	0,03044026		hsa-miR-145	-3,4033642	0,04645431	
	hsa-miR-542-5p	+54,34374	0,00590565		hsa-miR-638	-2,8906453	0,02154165	
	hsa-miR-18a	+30,91094	0,01265985		hsa-miR-572	-2,802281	0,04645431	
	hsa-miR-181c*	+13,449852	0,03186546		hsa-miR-2861	-2,7125058	0,02154165	
	hsa-miR-455-3p	+7,3237786	0,03868391		hsa-miR-140-3p	-2,6546035	0,04793501	
	hsa-miR-19b-1*	+6,336976	0,04645431		hsa-miR-29c	-2,1967037	0,0324926	
	hsa-miR-18b	+5,3216386	0,03186546		hsa-miR-3196	-2,0732105	0,04480261	
	hsa-miR-17	+4,3571143	0,04712037					
	hsa-miR-130a	+3,5983758	0,00481591					
	hsa-miR-106b	+3,255464	0,00936396					
	hsa-miR-19b	+3,2328632	0,0401878					
	hsa-miR-125a-5p	+3,0526762	0,04645431					
	hsa-miR-93	+2,5861104	0,00567414					

Tab. 7-4: Correlation matrix of all BCC and control samples (averaged values are shown in blue)

Group	Sample Name	1_control	2_control	3_control	4_control	5_control	6_control	7_control	1_BCC	2_BCC	3_BCC	4_BCC	5_BCC	6_BCC	7_BCC
control	1_control	1.000						0.929							0.914
	2_control	0.908	1.000												
	3_control	0.852	0.947	1.000											
	4_control	0.954	0.934	0.889	1.000										
	5_control	0.964	0.941	0.885	0.959	1.000									
	6_control	0.876	0.956	0.969	0.917	0.909	1.000								
	7_control	0.957	0.953	0.893	0.963	0.978	0.913	1.000							
BCC	1_BCC	0.944	0.909	0.862	0.963	0.938	0.889	0.940	1.000						0.952
	2_BCC	0.925	0.923	0.885	0.945	0.937	0.897	0.947	0.948	1.000					
	3_BCC	0.907	0.915	0.887	0.942	0.923	0.902	0.929	0.950	0.953	1.000				
	4_BCC	0.930	0.882	0.834	0.944	0.924	0.856	0.935	0.960	0.958	0.946	1.000			
	5_BCC	0.936	0.893	0.843	0.943	0.936	0.865	0.932	0.948	0.949	0.939	0.942	1.000		
	6_BCC	0.914	0.896	0.849	0.933	0.919	0.870	0.923	0.945	0.977	0.944	0.960	0.950	1.000	
	7_BCC	0.922	0.938	0.898	0.943	0.945	0.920	0.954	0.951	0.968	0.968	0.946	0.939	0.956	1.000

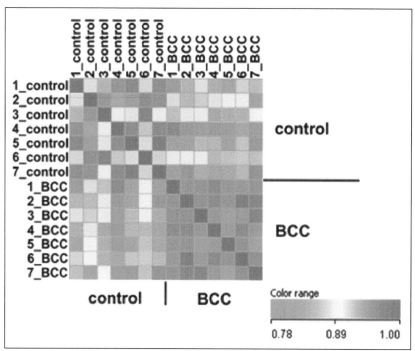

Fig. 7-1:   A heat map of the correlation coefficients r for the BCC and control groups is depicted. The color scale on the right side reflects the correlation of samples and runs from green (medium correlation) to red (high correlation). BCC= basal cell carcinoma

The MAPK/ERK pathway is involved in cell proliferation by activating transcription factors that result in DNA synthesis and mitosis. After the activation of membrane receptors, such as epidermal growth factor receptor (EGFR) or fibroblast growth factor receptor (FGFR), rat sarcoma (ras) family proteins (GTPases) trigger an intracellular kinase cascade that results in the phosphorylation of transcription factors by activated mitogen activated protein kinase (MAPK/ERK), thereby altering the cell cycle [13]. Parroo ct al. were the first to establish a direct connection between a cell signaling pathway implicated in the molecular pathogenesis of BCC and the miRNA machinery [14].

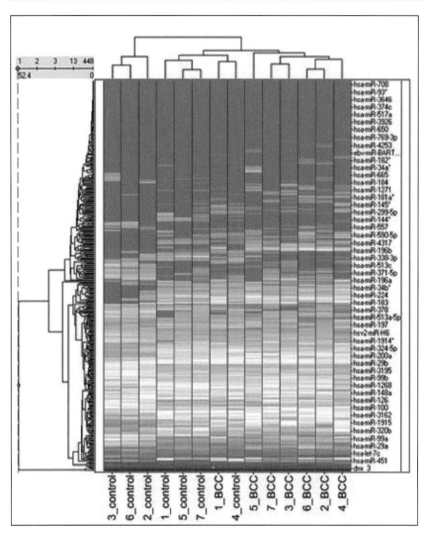

Fig. 7-2: The miRNA expression cluster analysis shows a strong similarity of the expression data in the heat map with 448 filtered miRNAs. The color scale reflects the log2 signal intensity and runs from red (low intensity) to white (medium intensity) to blue (strong intensity). The dendrogram on the left reflects the hierarchical similarity. The upper number in the scale above the dendrogram indicates the number of clusters at different positions in the dendrogram. The lower number is the similarity score for different positions in the dendrogram.

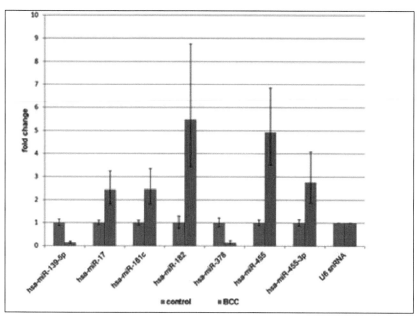

Fig. 7-3: The differential expression of up-regulated (hsa-miR-17, hsa-miR-181c, hsa-miR-455-3p, hsa-miR-455-5p, hsa-miR-182) and down-regulated (hsa-miR-378 and hsa-miR-139-5p) miRNAs in basal cell carcinoma (BCC) and control samples is graphed.

They established that the essential miRNA processing component TRBP (HIV-1 TAR RNA-binding protein), which is a co-factor of Dicer (a pivotal RNase III miRNA processing enzyme), is a target of MAPK/ERK phosphorylation. MAPK/ERK-mediated phosphorylation of TRBP stabilizes the miRNA processing complex, resulting in higher overall miRNA levels with an emphasis on the upregulation of pro-growth miRNAs and the downregulation of anti-growth miRNAs. The pro-growth miRNAs regulated *in vitro* by MAPK/ERK-induced phosphorylation of TRBP were hsa-miR-17, hsa-miR-20a and hsa-miR-92a [14]. In our set of differentially expressed miRNAs, hsa-miR-17 is one of the miRNAs that was significantly upregulated in BCC tissue (and validated by TaqMan qRT-PCR). The HH pathway, which has been shown to be essential for BCC proliferation and survival, is also linked to miRNA expression [15]. As a consequence of HH signaling, TGFbeta induction results in the downregulation of hsa-miR-141, hsa-miR-200a, hsa-miR-200b, hsa-miR-

200c, hsa-miR-205 and hsa-miR-429 [16]. HH signaling also activates protein patched homolog 1 (*PTCH*), the sonic hedgehog receptor. Mutations in *PTCH* are causative for Gorlin-Goltz syndrome (also known as basal cell nevus syndrome), and interestingly, *PTCH* is mutated in 30-67 % of spontaneous BCCs [2,17]. Medulloblastoma, the most common pediatric malignant brain tumor, has been associated with the diagnosis of Gorlin-Goltz syndrome and is defined as a minor criterion for its clinical diagnosis. Spontaneous medulloblastoma has a *PTCH* mutation rate of 10-20 % [18,19]. In addition, medulloblastoma has been associated with the hsa-miR-17-92 cluster, also known as Oncomir-1, which consists of 6 members (hsa-miR-17, hsa-miR-18a, hsa-miR-19a, hsa-miR-19b-1, hsa-miR-20a and hsa-miR-92) that are responsible for enhanced cell proliferation and the suppression of apoptosis [20,21]. Based on our preliminary data, which showed an up-regulation of hsa-miR-17, hsa-miR-18a, hsa-miR-18b (same seed sequence as hsa-miR-18a) and hsa-miR-19b-1 (consisting of hsa-miR-19-b and hsa-miR-19b-1*) in BCC (Tab. 7-3), we postulate that the hsa-miR-17-92 cluster collaborates with the Sonic Hedgehog pathway in both medulloblastoma and BCC [22]. The hsa-miR-17-92 cluster should therefore be further investigated in BCC.

Additional data mining revealed that *NOTCH4* and *KRAS* are target genes of hsa-miR-181c, which was up-regulated along with its opposite strand, hsa-miR-181c* [23]. *NOTCH* receptors and *KRAS* point mutations have previously been implicated in the pathogenesis of BCC [24,25]. Hsa-miR-182 has been linked to oncogenic transformation and has been described to negatively regulate human Forkhead-box O1 (*FOXO1*) expression in breast cancer cells [26]. Another member of the FOX family, human Forkhead-box M1 (*FOXM1*), is up-regulated in BCC by glioma transcription factor-1 (*Gli1*), which is a Sonic Hedgehog target [27,28].

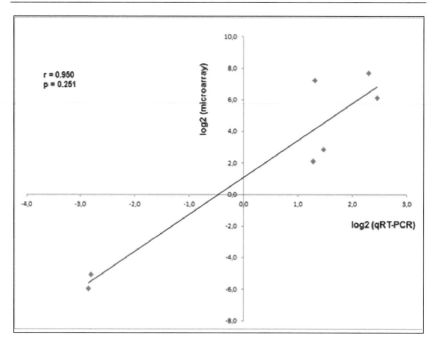

Fig. 7-4:   A scatter plot with a linear trend line of the qPCR and microarray results reveals no significant difference (p > 0.05) between the qRT-PCR and the microarray data (p=0.251). The results from these two assays were highly correlated (r= 0.95).

Whether hsa-miR-182 has a regulatory effect on *FOXM1*, as has been reported for *FOXO1*, cannot be confirmed based on available data but would be interesting to investigate. Similar to *FOXM1*, the promoter of the apoptosis regulator *BCL-2* can be activated by *GLI1* and *GLI2* in response to HH signaling in BCC [29]. *BCL-2* is predicted to be a target of hsa-miR-130a. The latter miRNA was significantly up-regulated in the BCC group in our data set. Therefore, it would be interesting to investigate a potential regulatory effect of hsa-miR-130a on *BCL-2*.

An interesting observation was made regarding the hsa-miR-106b-25 cluster, which consists of hsa-miR-106b, hsa-miR-93 and hsa-miR-25. It has been reported that the transcription factor *E2F1* is a target gene of hsa-miR-106b and hsa-miR-93 [30] as well as a transcriptional target of *GLI2* [31]. Increased *E2F1* activity contributes to BCC development in mice and suppresses epithelial apoptosis in humans[32,33]. Because hsa-miR-106b and hsa-miR-93 were both significantly up-regulated in our BCC cohort, we hypothesize that the hsa-miR-106b-25 cluster is involved in BCC pathogenesis and should be further investigated.

Elevated expression and activity of DNA methyltransferases (*DNMT*) *1*, *DNMT3A* and *DNMT3B* have been reported in UVB-exposed skin and UVB-induced skin tumors in mice [34]. Furthermore, it has been shown that the tumor suppressor genes *p16(INK4a)* and *RASSF1A* are transcriptionally silenced by hypermethylation [34]. Hsa-miR-29 was reported to down-regulate DNA methyltransferases *DNMT3A* and *DNMT3B* [35]. However, hsa-miR-29 and hsa-miR-29* were both signifi-cantly down-regulated in our BCC cohort, which would theoretically up-regulate *DNMT3A* and *DNMT3B*, resulting in increased DNA methylation that could silence tumor suppressor genes. Based on this preliminary evidence, it would be interesting to determine if UVB influences hsa-miR-29 levels and if down-regulated hsa-miR-29 is responsible for the hypermethylation-induced silencing of tumor suppressor genes that plays a role in the molecular pathogenesis of BCC.

Activation of type 1 insulin-like growth factor receptor (*IGF-1R*) signaling in basal epithelial cells led to spontaneous cutaneous tumor formation in a mouse model, in part by stimulating mitogenic pathways[36]. *IGF-1R* signaling has also been shown to synergize with SHH signaling in the granule cell precursors of the cerebellar cortex, which give rise to medulloblastoma [37]. Insulin receptor substrate-1 (*IRS-1*) activates *IGF-1R* and is an effector of Sonic Hedgehog signaling [38]. Hsa-miR-145, which was significantly down-regulated in our BCC cohort, has been proposed as a tumor suppressor that targets *IRS-1* in colon cancer cells[39]. Based on this preliminary data, the ability of hsa-miR-145 to downregulate the tumor suppressor *IRS-1* should be further investigated in BCC.

7.5   Conclusion

Based on preliminary microarray data, this study defines a set of miRNA candidates that should be considered for validation and functional examination as important mediators of the molecular pathogenesis of BCC.

7.6 Acknowledgements

The authors are grateful to Stefan Kotschote, MS and Dr. Cornelia Graf for technical advice.

7.7 References

1   Grimmer H. Histological picture report no.20l. Basalioma of the vulva (basal cell carcinoma Krompecher 1900). *Zeitschrift fur Haut und Geschlechtskrankheiten.* 1967; **43**:: 25-40.

2   Goppner D, Leverkus M. Basal cell carcinoma: from the molecular understanding of the pathogenesis to targeted therapy of progressive disease. *J Skin Cancer* 2011; **2011**: 650258.

3   Sand M, Gambichler T, Sand D *et al.* MicroRNAs and the skin: tiny players in the body's largest organ. *J Dermatol Sci* 2009; **53**: 169-75.

4   Sand M, Gambichler T, Skrygan M *et al.* Expression levels of the microRNA processing enzymes Drosha and dicer in epithelial skin cancer. *Cancer Invest* 2010; **28**: 649-53.

5   Sand M, Skrygan M, Georgas D *et al.* Expression levels of the microRNA maturing microprocessor complex component DGCR8 and the RNA-induced silencing complex (RISC) components Argonaute-1, Argonaute-2, PACT, TARBP1, and TARBP2 in epithelial skin cancer. *Mol Carcinog* 2011.

6   Zhang JD, Biczok R, Ruschhaupt M. The ddCt Algorithm for the Analysis of Quantitative Real-Time PCR (qRT-PCR). In. 2011.

7   Edgar R, Domrachev M, Lash AE. Gene Expression Omnibus: NCBI gene expression and hybridization array data repository. *Nucleic Acids Res* 2002; **30**: 207-10.

8   Sokal R, Michener C. A statistical method for evaluating systematic relationships. . *University of Kansas Science Bulletin* 1958; **38**:: 1409-38.

9   Quackenbush J. Computational analysis of microarray data. *Nat Rev Genet* 2001; **2**: 418-27.

10   Benjamini Y, Drai D, Elmer G *et al.* Controlling the false discovery rate in behavior genetics research. *Behav Brain Res* 2001; **125**: 279-84.

11   Jiang Q, Wang Y, Hao Y *et al.* miR2Disease: a manually curated database for microRNA deregulation in human disease. *Nucleic Acids Res* 2009; **37**: D98-104.

12   Epstein EH. Basal cell carcinomas: attack of the hedgehog. *Nat Rev Cancer* 2008; **8**: 743-54.

13   Johnson GL, Lapadat R. Mitogen-activated protein kinase pathways mediated by ERK, JNK, and p38 protein kinases. *Science* 2002; **298**: 1911-2.

14   Paroo Z, Ye X, Chen S *et al.* Phosphorylation of the human microRNA-generating complex mediates MAPK/Erk signaling. *Cell* 2009; **139**: 112-22.

15   Hutchin ME, Kariapper MS, Grachtchouk M *et al.* Sustained Hedgehog signaling is required for basal cell carcinoma proliferation and survival: conditional skin tumorigenesis recapitulates the hair growth cycle. *Genes Dev* 2005; **19**: 214-23.

16   Katoh Y, Katoh M. Hedgehog signaling, epithelial-to-mesenchymal transition and miRNA (review). *Int J Mol Med* 2008; **22**: 271-5.

17   Reifenberger J, Wolter M, Knobbe CB *et al.* Somatic mutations in the PTCH, SMOH, SUFUH and TP53 genes in sporadic basal cell carcinomas. *Br J Dermatol* 2005; **152**: 43-51.

18   Raffel C, Jenkins RB, Frederick L *et al.* Sporadic medulloblastomas contain PTCH mutations. *Cancer Res* 1997; **57**: 842-5.

19   Zurawel RH, Allen C, Chiappa S *et al.* Analysis of PTCH/SMO/SHH pathway genes in medulloblastoma. *Genes Chromosomes Cancer* 2000; **27**: 44-51.

20   He L, Thomson JM, Hemann MT *et al.* A microRNA polycistron as a potential human oncogene. *Nature* 2005; **435**: 828-33.

21   Al-Nakhle H, Burns PA, Cummings M *et al.* Estrogen receptor {beta}1 expression is regulated by miR-92 in breast cancer. *Cancer Res* 2010; **70**: 4778-84.

22 Uziel T, Karginov FV, Xie S *et al.* The miR-17~92 cluster collaborates with the Sonic Hedgehog pathway in medulloblastoma. *Proc Natl Acad Sci U S A* 2009; **106**: 2812-7.

23 Hashimoto Y, Akiyama Y, Otsubo T *et al.* Involvement of epigenetically silenced microRNA-181c in gastric carcinogenesis. *Carcinogenesis* 2010; **31**: 777-84.

24 Proweller A, Tu L, Lepore JJ *et al.* Impaired notch signaling promotes de novo squamous cell carcinoma formation. *Cancer Res* 2006; **66**: 7438-44.

25 van der Schroeff JG, Evers LM, Boot AJ *et al.* Ras oncogene mutations in basal cell carcinomas and squamous cell carcinomas of human skin. *J Invest Dermatol* 1990; **94**: 423-5.

26 Guttilla IK, White BA. Coordinate regulation of FOXO1 by miR-27a, miR-96, and miR-182 in breast cancer cells. *J Biol Chem* 2009; **284**: 23204-16.

27 Katoh M. Human FOX gene family (Review). *Int J Oncol* 2004; **25**: 1495-500.

28 Teh MT, Wong ST, Neill GW *et al.* FOXM1 is a downstream target of Gli1 in basal cell carcinomas. *Cancer Res* 2002; **62**: 4773-80.

29 Regl G, Kasper M, Schnidar H *et al.* Activation of the BCL2 promoter in response to Hedgehog/GLI signal transduction is predominantly mediated by GLI2. *Cancer Res* 2004; **64**: 7724-31.

30 Li Y, Tan W, Neo TW *et al.* Role of the miR-106b-25 microRNA cluster in hepatocellular carcinoma. *Cancer Sci* 2009; **100**: 1234-42.

31 Regl G, Kasper M, Schnidar H *et al.* The zinc-finger transcription factor GLI2 antagonizes contact inhibition and differentiation of human epidermal cells. *Oncogene* 2004; **23**: 1263-74.

32 Pierce AM, Gimenez-Conti IB, Schneider-Broussard R *et al.* Increased E2F1 activity induces skin tumors in mice heterozygous and nullizygous for p53. *Proc Natl Acad Sci U S A* 1998; **95**: 8858-63.

33 Berton TR, Mitchell DL, Guo R *et al.* Regulation of epidermal apoptosis and DNA repair by E2F1 in response to ultraviolet B radiation. *Oncogene* 2005; **24**: 2449-60.

34   Nandakumar V, Vaid M, Tollefsbol TO *et al.* Aberrant DNA hypermethylation patterns lead to transcriptional silencing of tumor suppressor genes in UVB-exposed skin and UVB-induced skin tumors of mice. *Carcinogenesis* 2011; **32**: 597-604.

35   Nguyen T, Kuo C, Nicholl MB *et al.* Downregulation of microRNA-29c is associated with hypermethylation of tumor-related genes and disease outcome in cutaneous melanoma. *Epigenetics* 2011; **6**: 388-94.

36   DiGiovanni J, Bol DK, Wilker E *et al.* Constitutive expression of insulin-like growth factor-1 in epidermal basal cells of transgenic mice leads to spontaneous tumor promotion. *Cancer Res* 2000; **60**: 1561-70.

37   Fernandez C, Tatard VM, Bertrand N *et al.* Differential modulation of Sonic-hedgehog-induced cerebellar granule cell precursor proliferation by the IGF signaling network. *Dev Neurosci* 2010; **32**: 59-70.

38   Parathath SR, Mainwaring LA, Fernandez LA *et al.* Insulin receptor substrate 1 is an effector of sonic hedgehog mitogenic signaling in cerebellar neural precursors. *Development* 2008; **135**: 3291-300.

39   Shi B, Sepp-Lorenzino L, Prisco M *et al.* Micro RNA 145 targets the insulin receptor substrate-1 and inhibits the growth of colon cancer cells. *J Biol Chem* 2007; **282**: 32582-90.

8 Paper 4: Microarray analysis of microRNA expression in cutaneous squamous cell carcinoma*

8.1 Introduction

MicroRNAs (miRNAs) are a relatively new class of non-coding RNA molecules. They are 17-21 nucleotides (nt) in length and are capable of post-transcriptional gene silencing [1]. Pri-miRNAs are transcribed in the nucleus by RNA polymerases II and III before being processed by the miRNA maturing enzymes, Drosha (intranuclear) and Dicer (extranuclear). The latter enzyme is also part of the RNA-induced silencing complex (RISC), which regulates gene function once the mature miRNA has been loaded onto it. After Watson-Crick base pairing occurs between the target mRNA and the 5' "seed region" of the RISC-loaded miRNA, the target mRNA will either be translationally repressed (in the case of weak mRNA/miRNA complementarity) or be cleaved (in the case of strong mRNA/miRNA complementarity) causing posttranscriptional gene silencing [2]. Despite the significant potential for miRNA-based therapy, little research has been performed on miRNA roles in cutaneous squamous cell carcinoma (cSCC).

In two recent studies, we were able to show dysregulation of the expression of Dicer, Drosha and the RISC components in cSCC [3, 4]. Several other studies have shown perturbations of miRNA expression in different forms of cancer, including cervical, lung, esophageal, oral, pharyngeal and tongue squamous cell carcinoma[5-9]. Although a small group of specific miRNAs that were previously described in keratinocytes has been investigated in cSCC via real-time reverse transcriptase-PCR analysis, thus far, no research has focused on global microarray miRNA expression profiling in cSCC [10, 11]. Preliminary findings have suggested that perturbations in the miRNA machinery exist in cSCC like they have recently been shown in basal cell carcinoma; therefore, this study was performed to identify potentially dysregulated miRNAs in cSCC using microarray-based miRNA expression profiling[12].

---

* Co-authors: Marina Skrygan Ph.D., Dimitrios Georgas M.D., Daniel Sand M.D., Stephan A. Hahn M.D., Thilo Gambichler M.D., Peter Altmeyer M.D., Falk G. Bechara M.D.

8.2   Materials and Methods

The present study was approved by the Ethical Review Board of the Ruhr-University Bochum, Germany (registration number: 3265-08, ClinicalTrials.gov Identifier: NCT01500954). Furthermore, it was conducted within the framework of the declaration of Helsinki, and informed consent forms were signed by all study subjects.
Subjects

In 7 patients (3 females, 4 males; median age: 80.3 years), biopsy specimens of cSCC and control specimens from an adjacent healthy skin site near the tumor border (intraindividual control) were obtained during surgical removal of the tumor (Tab. 8-1). Specimens were immediately stored in RNAlater (Qiagen, Hilden, Germany) at -80 °C.

8.2.1   RNA isolation

Total RNA, including miRNA, was isolated with the miRNeasy Mini Kit (Quiagen, Hilden, Germany) according to the manufacturer's protocol. For RNA quality control purposes, we determined the RNA concentration, purity and RNA integrity number (RIN) using the Agilent 2100 Bioanalyzer, the RNA 6000 Nano LabCHip Kits (both Agilent Technologies, Santa Clara, USA) and the NanoDrop ND-1000 spectral photometer (Peqlab, Erlangen, Germany). We defined a RIN $\geq$ 6.7 as a minimal inclusion criterion to be acceptable for further microarray analysis.

8.2.2   Preparation of labeled miRNA, microarray hybridization and scanning

All of the following steps were performed according to the manufacturer´s protocol. To assess the labeling and hybridization efficiencies, total RNA samples were spiked with MicroRNA Spike-In Kit (Agilent Technologies, Santa Clara, USA). After treatment with calf intestine phosphatase (CIP), a labeling reaction was initiated with 100 ng total RNA per sample. For labeling dephosphorylated RNA, a T4 RNA ligase that incorporates cyanine 3-cytidine bisphosphate (miRNA Complete Labeling and Hyb Kit, Agilent Technologies, Santa Clara, USA) was used. The cyanine-3-labeled miRNA samples were then prepared for One-Color-based hybridization (Complete miRNA Labeling and Hyb Kit, Agilent Technologies, Santa Clara, USA). Hybridization was performed at 55°C for 20 hrs on human miRNA Microarrays Release 16.0, 8x60K format (Agilent Technologies, Santa Clara, USA). The microarray slides were washed (Gene Expression Wash Buffers, Agilent Technologies, Santa Clara, USA) and dried with acetonitrile (Sigma-Aldrich, St. Louis, USA). Fluorescent signal intensities were detected with an Agilent DNA Microarray Scanner (Agilent Technologies, Santa Clara, USA) and Scan Control A.8.4.1 Software (Agilent Technologies, Santa Clara, USA). The data were extracted using Feature Extraction 10.7.3.1 Software (Agilent Technologies, Santa Clara, USA).

8.2.3   *TaqMan quantitative real-time reverse transcription polymerase chain reaction (qRT-PCR)*

TaqMan qRT-PCR was used to validate the microarray data. TaqMan MicroRNA assays (Applied Biosystems, Darmstadt, Germany) for four up-regulated miRNAs, three down-regulated miRNAs and the reference gene snRNA U6 were used for TaqMan quantitative real-time reverse transcription polymerase chain reactions (qRT-PCRs).

TaqMan qRT-PCR analysis was performed according to the manufacturer's instructions. The TaqMan MicroRNA Reverse Transcription Kit (Applied Biosystems, Darmstadt, Germany) was used to reverse transcribe a miRNA into single-stranded cDNA with the aid of assay-specific primers according to the manufacturer's instructions. Ten nanograms of total RNA was reverse transcribed from each sample of analyzed miRNA. qPCR analysis was conducted in technical replicates according to the manufacturer's instructions using the TaqMan Universal MasterMix II no UNG (Applied Biosystems, Darmstadt, Germany) in a final reaction volume of 10 µl. The reaction mix was transferred into 384-well plates and run on an AB7900HT instrument (Applied Biosystems, Darmstadt, Germany). The software *SDS 2.4* (Applied Biosystems, Darmstadt, Germany) was used for instrument control, data acquisition and raw data analysis. The analyses were performed in Relative Quantification ($\Delta\Delta C_t$) mode with triplicate measurements. The following temperature profile was used: 50°C / 2:00 min – 95°C / 10:00 min – 40 cycles x [95°C / 0:15 min – 60°C / 1:00 min]. The $\Delta\Delta C_t$ method as previously described by Zhang et al. was applied to calculate the relative expression levels of the target miRNAs [13]. Fold-change values of the selected miRNAs were transformed to $\log_2$ values, both for qRT-PCR and for microarray results. To compare the data from the qRT-PCR and microarray analyses, a paired two-sample t-test (significance level set at $p < 0.05$) and Pearson´s correlation coefficient r were calculated based on $\log_2$ values.

8.2.4   Bioinformatic Data analyses

The data discussed in this study have been deposited in NCBI's Gene Expression Omnibus (GEO) and are accessible through GEO Series accession number GSE34536 (Internet address: http://www.ncbi.nlm.nih. gov/geo/query/acc.cgi? acc=GSE34536) [14]. Feature Extraction 10.7.3.1 and GeneSpring GX 11.5.1 software (both Agilent Technologies, Santa Clara, USA) were used for quality control, statistical data analysis, miRNA annotation and visualization. For equal distribution of probe signal intensities, quantile normalization was applied to the data set. We applied the Unweighted Pair-Group Method with Arithmetic mean (UPGMA) based on Euclidian distance to normalized data to perform a hierarchical clustering analysis [15, 16]. Pearson's correlation coefficients (r) were calculated for every specimen within the two groups and for pair-wise comparison. Normalized and $\log_2$ transformed data were averaged across the replicates. The following pair-wise comparisons were analyzed: the non-lesional epithelial skin (control) was used as a reference group, and cSCC was compared to this baseline.

Tab. 8-1: Details of BCC and control specimen.
mm=millimeters, BCC= basal cell carcinoma, RIN= RNA integrity number. n.a.= not applicable

Sample ID	Sex	Age	Localisation	Histology	Invasion depth	RNA conc. (ng/µl)	A260/280 ratio	RIN
1_SCC	m	78	Hand	SCC, highly differentiated CL III-IV, G2	3.4 mm	165.94	2.02	8.2
1_control	m	78	Hand	non-lesional epithelial skin	n.a.	29.90	1.69	9.3
2_SCC	m	86	Helix	SCC, highly differentiated CL IV, G1	6.2 mm	887.95	2.09	9.0
2_control	m	86	Helix	non-lesional epithelial skin	n.a.	98.26	1.93	7.2
3_SCC	m	74	Scalp	SCC, highly differentiated CL IV, G2	4.3 mm	876.87	2.09	8.9
3_control	m	74	Scalp	non-lesional epithelial skin	n.a.	96.60	1.85	9.1
4_SCC	w	82	Cheek	SCC, good differentiated CL V, G1	8.4 mm	330.93	2.03	9.0
4_control	w	82	Cheek	non-lesional epithelial skin	n.a.	63.95	1.97	8.6

Tab. 8-1:   (Continued)

Sample ID	Sex	Age	Localisation	Histology	Invasion depth	RNA conc. (ng/ µl)	A260/280 raio	RIN
5_SCC	m	66	Scalp	SCC highly differentiated CL IV, G1	3.1 mm	301.64	2.00	8.0
5_control	m	66	Scalp	non-lesional epithelial skin	n.a.	48.60	1.76	7.9
6_SCC	w	90	Forehead	SCC highly differentiated CL IV-V, G1	7 mm	280.47	2.04	8.2
6_control	w	90	Forehead	non-lesional epithelial skin	n.a.	26.59	1.75	6.7
7_SCC	w	86	Lower lip	SCC highly differentiated CL IV, G1	2.9 mm	207.18	2.05	8.2
7_control	w	86	Lower lip	non-lesional epithelial skin	n.a.	33.23	2.11	8.3

8.2.5   Statistical analyses

Different groups were compared by applying a paired t-test with an adjusted p-value.

The algorithm devised by Benjamini and Hochberg was applied to calculate the adjusted p-value [17]. For comparison, the two groups (cSCC and control) were compared in a pairwise manner. A fold-change value was calculated to determine the extent and direction of differential expression between cSCC and the control. Therefore, normalized signal values were transformed from $\log^2$ to a linear scale. Statistical significance and robust detection were evaluated to identify differentially expressed miRNAs. Two different p values were defined depending on a stringent or a non-stringent filtering approach in the comparison of cSCC and the control. Applying the non-stringent filtering approach, a probe was defined as induced if its non-adjusted p-value was $\leq$ 0.01 and 0.05 with a fold-change value $\geq$ 2.0 and repressed if its non-adjusted p-value was $\leq$ 0.01 and 0.05 with a fold-change value $\geq$ - 2.0. Applying the stringent filtering approach, a probe was classified as induced when the corrected p-value was $\leq$ 0.05 with a fold-change value $\geq$ 2.0 and as repressed if its corrected p-value was $\leq$ 0.05 with a fold-change value $\geq$ - 2.0.

8.2.6   Mining Data Analysis

To evaluate the list of differentially expressed miRNAs in the context of the current literature, we performed a systematic mining data analysis. The following databases and miRNA target prediction sites were utilized: miRNA database for miRNA functional annotations miRDB (http://mirdb.org/miRDB), Target Scan Human for predicting miRNA targets (http://www.targetscan.org/), miRò miRNA knowledge base (http://ferrolab.dmi.unict.it/miro), Mir2Disease database (http://www.mir2 disease.org/)[18], the human miRNA-associated disease database HMDD (http://cmbi.bjmu.edu.cn/hmdd), the miRNA database miRBase (http://www.mirbase.org) and PubMed (http://www.ncbi.nlm.nih.gov/ pubmed/).

Tab. 8-2: Correlation matrix of SCC and control samples (averaged values are shown in blue)

Group	Sample Name	1_control	2_control	3_control	4_control	5_control	6_control	7_control	1_SCC	2_SCC	3_SCC	4_SCC	5_SCC	6_SCC	7_SCC
Control	1_control	1.000						0.923							0.903
	2_control	0.861	1.000												
	3_control	0.892	0.978	1.000											
	4_control	0.857	0.988	0.969	1.000										
	5_control	0.940	0.899	0.919	0.896	1.000									
	6_control	0.924	0.924	0.939	0.928	0.933	1.000								
	7_control	0.889	0.937	0.942	0.932	0.901	0.940	1.000							
SCC	1_SCC	0.850	0.934	0.937	0.937	0.855	0.912	0.932	1.000						0.899
	2_SCC	0.880	0.934	0.939	0.941	0.890	0.924	0.910	0.930	1.000					
	3_SCC	0.823	0.930	0.933	0.925	0.836	0.886	0.887	0.933	0.934	1.000				
	4_SCC	0.863	0.943	0.945	0.936	0.864	0.908	0.919	0.952	0.933	0.941	1.000			
	5_SCC	0.903	0.944	0.956	0.926	0.910	0.923	0.922	0.923	0.920	0.907	0.955	1.000		
	6_SCC	0.942	0.790	0.824	0.784	0.886	0.854	0.812	0.786	0.827	0.767	0.809	0.868	1.000	
	7_SCC	0.877	0.948	0.955	0.944	0.888	0.929	0.955	0.947	0.930	0.917	0.940	0.936	0.815	1.000

8.3   Results

8.3.1   Quality control

Quality control (QC) reports were generated for each microarray with Feature Extraction software 10.7.3.1 (Agilent Technologies, Santa Clara, USA). All QC reports showed that all quality criteria for successful microarray analysis were met as pre-defined by the microarray manufacturer. Correct automatic corner finding and grid placing were confirmed by visually monitoring the corner spots.

8.3.2   Differential miRNA expression

With the non-stringent filtering approach, we found thirteen up-regulated and eighteen down-regulated miRNAs in cSCC (non-adjusted $p \leq 0.05$). For details, see Tab. 8-4. By applying the non-stringent filtering approach (non-adjusted $p \leq 0.01$), however, we found three up-regulated (hsa-miR-135b, hsa-miR-424 and hsa-miR-766) and six down-regulated (hsa-miR-30a*, hsa-miR-378, hsa-miR-145, hsa-miR-140-3p, hsa-miR-30a and hsa-miR-26a) miRNAs in cutaneous SCC. By applying the stringent filtering approach (adjusted $p \leq 0.05$) we could not define significant up- or down regulation.

8.3.3   Correlation analysis

A correlation analysis revealed medium to high correlation between and within each group as expressed in the Pearson's correlation coefficient r. R ranged from 0.857 to 0.988 with an average r of 0.923 within the control group, whereas R ranged from 0.767 to 0.955 with an average r of 0.899 within the SCC group. The correlation coefficients and controls ranged from 0.784 to 0.956 with an average r of 0.903. Tab. 8-2 and Fig. 8-1 summarize the findings of the correlation analysis.

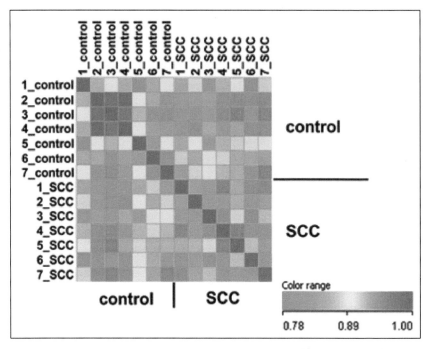

Fig. 8-1:   Correlation coefficients r for cutaneous squamous cell carcinoma (cSCC) and control samples. The color scale on the right shows the correlation of samples and runs from green, reflecting medium correlation, to red, reflecting high correlation. SCC=squamous cell carcinoma

8.3.4   Cluster analysis

The heat map generated for cluster analysis showed heterogeneous miRNA expression profiles with a maximum of three specimens of the same group per cluster (1_SCC, 4_SCC, 5_SCC and 3_control, 2_control, 4_control). Overall, we observed a high degree of similarity between cSCC and the control, which was expected because we were analyzing biological replicates of the same tissue type [Fig. 8-2].

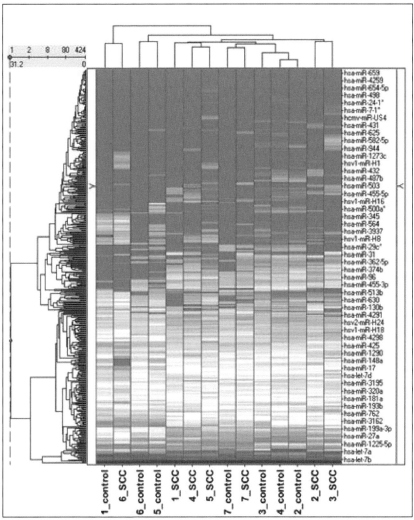

Fig. 8-2: Heat-map of cSCC and control miRNA expression illustrating cluster analysis of the expression data of 424 filtered miRNAs showing a high degree of similarity. The signal intensity converted to log2 is reflected in the color scale such that red, white and blue show low, medium and strong miRNA expression, respectively. The dendrogram on the left reflects hierarchical similarity. The upper number in the scale above the dendrogram shows the number of clusters at different positions in the dendrogram. The lower number shows the similarity score for different positions in the dendrogram.

8.3.5   TaqMan RT-PCR Validation

Microarray results were validated by means of TaqMan qRT-PCR expression analysis of the following miRNAs, which were calculated to be differentially expressed according to a previous microarray analysis: hsa-miR-31, hsa-miR-135b, hsa-miR-424, and hsa-miR-21 (up-regulated) and hsa-miR-30a, hsa-miR-30a* and hsa-miR-378 (down-regulated).

The qRT-PCR results of these target miRNAs are compiled in Fig. 8-3. Pearson´s correlation coefficient r= 0.978 showed a high degree of correlation. The p value based on a paired two-sample t-test was p= 0.824 (p > 0.05), which shows that there is no significant difference between the qRT-PCR and microarray results for the examined miRNAs (Fig. 8-4).

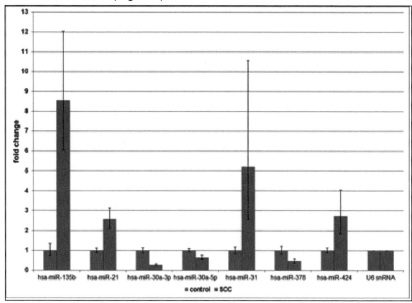

Fig. 8-3:   Differential expression of up-regulated (hsa-miR-31, hsa-miR-135b, hsa-miR-424, hsa-miR-21) and down-regulated (hsa-miR-30a, hsa-miR-30a* and hsa-miR-378) miRNAs in squamous cell carcinoma (SCC) and control.

8.3.6   Mining data analysis results

The results and discussion of the mining data analysis are compiled in the next section.

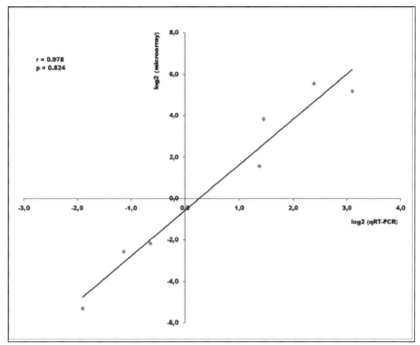

Fig. 8-4:   qPCR and microarray results as a scatter plot with a linear trend line. There was no significant difference between qRT-PCR and microarray data (p=0.824; p > 0.05). Microarray and qRT-PCR results showed a high degree of correlation (r= 0.978).

8.4   Discussion

After basal cell carcinoma (BCC), cutaneous SCC (cSCC) is the second most common type of epithelial skin cancer and accounts for 20 % of all skin cancer–related deaths[19]. cSCC originates from the malignant proliferation of epidermal keratinocytes. Differential mRNA expression profiling for cSCC using cDNA microarrays has revealed a variety of genes that are dysregulated in cSCC compared to healthy skin[20]. However, miRNA expression profiling in multiple human cancers has been shown to be more accurate with regards to tumor classification compared to mRNA expression profiling [21, 22]. Whether this trend is also true for cSCC has not yet been investigated.

Preliminary findings have shown that the miRNA machinery is perturbed in cSCC[3, 4]. Additionally, the dysregulation in miRNA expression profiles has been described for a variety of different SCCs, though not for cSCC. Therefore, the next necessary step was to perform a global miRNA expression profiling study to describe specific, potentially dysregulated miRNAs in cSCC. The present cSCC miRNA profiling study is based on miRBase 16 and scanned for 1205 human miRNAs on the microarray chip.

Dziunycz et al. were the first to examine a group of selected miRNAs in cSCC that were previously described to have a function in keratinocytes[11]. Based on a real-time reverse transcriptase-PCR analysis, they investigated hsa-miR-21, hsa-miR-184, hsa-miR-203 and hsa-miR-205 in cSCC of immunocompetent subjects and organ transplant recipients. These authors showed that hsa-miR-21 and hsa-miR-184 expression was significantly increased and that hsa-miR-203 expression was significantly decreased in cSCC compared to normal skin. Based on our data set, we were able to confirm that hsa-miR-21 and hsa-miR-21* were overexpressed. Hsa-miR-21 has been extensively studied in a variety of cancers, including non-cutaneous SCC, oral and esophageal SCC and laryngeal cancer [23-25]. UV-A irradiation of skin keratinocytes has been shown to result in hsa-miR-21 overexpression, whereas UV-B irradiation had little to no effect on its expression [11]. Reversion-inducing cysteine-rich protein with Kazal motifs (RECK) and tissue inhibitor of metalloproteinase 3 (Timp3), which are both tumor suppressors and inhibitors of matrix metalloproteinases (MMPs), as well as tumor suppressor programmed cell death 4 (PDCD4) and tropomyosin 1 (TPM1) have been shown to be down-regulated by hsa-miR-21 [26-28]. RECK and Timp3 down-regulation has also been shown in squamous cell lung cancer, and there is evidence for PDCD4 down-regulation in cSCC in a transgenic mouse model and for hsa-miR-21 mediated TPM1 down-regulation in tongue SCC [9, 27, 29, 30]. This preliminary evidence suggests that it would be interesting to investigate whether hsa-miR-21 induced down-regulation of RECK, Timp3, PDCD4 or TPM1 could be confirmed in cSCC.

Tab. 8-3: Comparison of SCC vs. control with stringent (adjusted-p ≤ 0.05) and non-stringent (p ≤ 0.01) filtering. Significantly up- and down-regulated miRNAs are sorted by their FC. FC= fold change, SCC= squamous cell carcinoma

Comparison	adj.-p ≤ 0.05 $|FC| ≥ 2.0$ Up	adj.-p ≤ 0.05 $|FC| ≥ 2.0$ Down	p ≤ 0.01 $|FC| ≥ 2.0$ Up	p ≤ 0.01 $|FC| ≥ 2.0$ Down	miRNA	Fold change	p-value
SCC_tumor vs. SCC_normal	0	0	3	6			
SCC_tumor vs. SCC_normal (miRNA detail) Up	0	0			hsa-miR-135b	+36.243248	0.009520266
					hsa-miR-424	+14.225932	0.006567399
					hsa-miR-766	+6.6804285	0.006159176
SCC_tumor vs. SCC_normal (miRNA detail) Down	0	0			hsa-miR-30a*	-39.39772	0.001121986
					hsa-miR-378	-5.9355726	0.002162511
					hsa-miR-145	-3.682301	0.001721313
					hsa-miR-140-3p	-2.459666	0.005457281
					hsa-miR-30a	-4.4591885	0.001027054
					hsa-miR-26a	-2.1028998	0.005589837

Tab. 8-4: Comparison of SCC vs. control with non-stringent filtering (p ≤ 0.05). Significantly up- and down-regulated miRNAs are sorted by their FC. FC= fold change, SCC= squamous cell carcinoma

Comparison	p ≤ 0.05 $|FC| ≥ 2.0$			
SCC_tumor vs. SCC_normal	Up	13		
		miRNA	**Fold change**	**p-value**
SCC_tumor vs. SCC_normal (miRNA detail)		hsa-miR-31	+47.025654	0.02327827
		hsa-miR-135b	+36.243248	0.009520266
		hsa-miR-31*	+19.058601	0.03265999
		hsa-miR-424	+14.225932	0.006567399
		hsa-miR-21*	+13.862657	0.023449535
		hsa-miR-374a	+9.915963	0.037786435
		hsa-miR-196a	+7.338848	0.03689442
		hsa-miR-18a	+6.6910186	0.029686995
		hsa-miR-766	+6.6804285	0.0061159176
		hsa-miR-128	+5.9752536	0.04759205
		hsa-miR-130b	+5.682557	0.02480776
		hsa-miR-455-5p	+4.4701114	0.047512535
		hsa-miR-21	+2.977366	0.015169031

Tab. 8-4:   (Continued)

Comparison	p ≤ 0.05 |FC| ≥ 2.0			
	Down			
	18			
	miRNA	Fold change	p-value	
SCC_tumor vs. SCC_normal	hsa-miR-30a*	-39.39772	0.001121986	
	hsa-miR-133b	-19.919054	0.045951728	
	hsa-miR-101	-17.007914	0.013958397	
	hsa-miR-4324	-10.5915365	0.014990797	
	hsa-miR-136	-6.587424	0.015773607	
	hsa-miR-378	-5.9355726	0.002162511	
SCC_tumor vs. SCC_normal (miRNA detail)	hsa-miR-30a	-4.4591885	0.001027054	
	hsa-miR-204	-4.4122844	0.03805398	
	hsa-miR-497	-4.3927507	0.015091389	
	hsa-miR-378*	-4.2924438	0.032041933	
	hsa-miR-29c*	-4.2608275	0.04898456	
	hsa-miR-214	-4.2438507	0.020694578	
	hsa-miR-145	-3.682301	0.001721313	
	hsa-miR-199a-5p	-3.4887564	0.023821056	
	hsa-miR-125b	-2.8608308	0.03838354	
	hsa-miR-140-3p	-2.459666	0.005457281	
	hsa-miR-125b-2*	-2.2649415	0.023497948	
	hsa-miR-26a	-2.1028998	0.005589837	

Tab. 8-5: Molecular impact of significantly (p ≤ 0.01) up- and down-regulated miRNAs in cSCC.

miRNA	Regu-lation	Molecular Impact	Author Molecular Impact
hsa-miR-135b	+	Biomarker for pancreatic ductal adenocarcinoma, mediates oncogenicity in anaplastic large cell lymphoma	Munding et al. [42] Matsuyama et al. [43]
hsa-miR-424	+	Promotes angiogenesis, regulates cell-autonomous angiogenic functions	Ghosh et al.[44] Chamorro-Jorganes et al. [45]
hsa-miR-766	+	n.a.	
hsa-miR-26a	-	Downregulation of oncogene Histone-lysine N-methyltransferase (EZH2)	Lu et al. [46] Sander et al. [47]
hsa-miR-30a	-	Inhibits epithelial-to-mesenchymal transition, an essential component of cancer metastasis and progression by targeting Snai1 and is downregulated in non-small cell lung cancer; surpresses tumor growth in colon carcinoma by targeting denticleless protein homolog (DTL)	Kumarswamy et al. [48] Baraniskin et al. [49]
hsa-miR-30a*	-	n.a.	
hsa-miR-140-3p	-	Targets CD38; down-regulated in basal cell carcinoma	Jude et al. [50] Sand et al. [12]
hsa-miR-145	-	Inhibits actin-binding protein Fascin homolog 1 (FSCN1) in esophageal squamous cell carcinoma; down-regulated in basal cell carcinoma	Kano et al. [51] Sand et al. [12]
hsa-miR-378	-	Targets insulin-like growth factor 1 receptor (IGF1R) and caspase 3; down-regulated in basal cell carcinoma	Knezevic et al. [52] Fang et al. [53] Sand et al. [12]

Hsa-miR-18a is part of the hsa-miR-17-92 cluster also known as Oncomir-1, a polycistronic miRNA that consists of hsa-miR-17, hsa-miR-18a, hsa-miR-19a, hsa-miR-19b-1, hsa-miR20a and hsa-miR-92 [31].

The hsa-miR-17-92 cluster has been shown to cooperate with the Sonic Hedgehog pathway in medulloblastoma [32]. Hedgehog (Hh) signaling has also been linked to the molecular pathogenesis of cSCC [33]. The potential for hsa-miR-18a-mediated interference with Hh signaling in cSCC should be further investigated. Hsa-miR-128a, which is inversely related to IL-17 and IL-4 in human breast cancer, is another miRNA candidate for further analysis, as it has been shown that IL-4 mediates the apoptotic pathway in oral SCC, indicating a possible role in cSCC [34, 35]. As has been previously shown, the tumor suppressor tumor protein 53-induced nuclear protein 1 (TP53INP1) is down-regulated by hsa-miR-130b [36]. As this miRNA was significantly up-regulated, it would be interesting to examine whether the hsa-miR-130b / TP53INP1-axis could be reproduced for cSCC. Furthermore, dysregulation of the oncogene pyruvate kinase type M2 (PKM2) by hsa-miR-133b has been shown in tongue SCC cell lines [37]. As hsa-miR-133b was significantly down-regulated in our cSCC group, whether hsa-miR-133b-mediated PKM2 dysregulation occurs in cSCC should be further investigated.

Hsa-miR-101 down-regulation has been observed in a variety of different cancers such as bladder cancer, hepatocellular carcinoma, lung cancer, prostate cancer and, in our study, cSCC. At the same time, hsa-miR-101 has shown to target and significantly repress myeloid cell leukemia-1 (Mcl-1) [38]. Promising results have been reported for the inhibition of Mcl-1 by siRNA in human oral SCC [39]. Whether hsa-miR-101-mediated Mcl-1 inhibition would result in cell growth inhibition of cSCC remains to be determined. Hsa-miR-204 has previously been described as down-regulated in oral SCC and as a tumor suppressor in SCC of the head and neck [40, 41]. As hsa-miR-204 was also down-regulated in cSCC in our study, hsa-miR-204 could be an interesting candidate for further analysis.

In the present miRNA profiling study for cSCC we have defined several p values for data analysis (Tab. 8-3 and Tab. 8-4). The original p-value was defined as $p \leq 0.01$ and $p \leq 0.05$. Additionally we have applied a correction to the original p-value as the number of hypotheses (= probes on the microarray) is much higher than the number of analyzed samples. A well-established method for this adjustment is the algorithm devised by Benjamini and Hochberg, which is based on a control of the false discovery rate (FDR) [17]. The p-value adjusted for multiple testing is usually several orders of magnitude higher than the unadjusted p-value. However the most significant findings were achieved with the original p-value ≤ 0.01 which resulted in three significantly up- and nine significantly down-regulated miRNAs ($p \leq 0.01$).

The most important molecular impacts of this differentially expressed miRNAs are compiled in Tab. 8-5.

This microarray-based, genome-wide miRNA profiling study revealed a list of differentially expressed miRNA candidates in cSCC that should be validated and analyzed for their involvement in the molecular pathogenesis of this disease.

8.5   Acknowledgements

The authors are grateful to Dr. Cornelia Graf and Stefan Kotschote, MS, for technical advice.

8.6   References

[1] Sand M, Gambichler T, Sand D, Skrygan M, Altmeyer P, Bechara FG: MicroRNAs and the skin: tiny players in the body's largest organ. J Dermatol Sci 53: 169-175, 2009.

[2] Grimson A, Farh KK, Johnston WK, Garrett-Engele P, Lim LP, Bartel DP: MicroRNA targeting specificity in mammals: determinants beyond seed pairing. Mol Cell 27: 91-105, 2007.

[3] Sand M, Gambichler T, Skrygan M, Sand D, Scola N, Altmeyer P, et al.: Expression levels of the microRNA processing enzymes Drosha and dicer in epithelial skin cancer. Cancer Invest 28: 649-653, 2010.

[4] Sand M, Skrygan M, Georgas D, Arenz C, Gambichler T, Sand D, et al.: Expression levels of the microRNA maturing microprocessor complex component DGCR8 and the RNA-induced silencing complex (RISC) components Argonaute-1, Argonaute-2, PACT, TARBP1, and TARBP2 in epithelial skin cancer. Mol Carcinog, 2011.

[5] Muralidhar B, Winder D, Murray M, Palmer R, Barbosa-Morais N, Saini H, et al.: Functional evidence that Drosha overexpression in cervical squamous cell carcinoma affects cell phenotype and microRNA profiles. J Pathol 224: 496-507, 2011.

[6] Yang Y, Li X, Yang Q, Wang X, Zhou Y, Jiang T, et al.: The role of microRNA in human lung squamous cell carcinoma. Cancer Genet Cytogenet 200: 127-133, 2010.

[7] Mathe EA, Nguyen GH, Bowman ED, Zhao Y, Budhu A, Schetter AJ, et al.: MicroRNA expression in squamous cell carcinoma and adenocarcinoma of the esophagus: associations with survival. Clin Cancer Res 15: 6192-6200, 2009.

[8] Lajer CB, Nielsen FC, Friis-Hansen L, Norrild B, Borup R, Garnaes E, et al.: Different miRNA signatures of oral and pharyngeal squamous cell carcinomas: a prospective translational study. Br J Cancer 104: 830-840, 2011.

[9] Li J, Huang H, Sun L, Yang M, Pan C, Chen W, et al.: MiR-21 indicates poor prognosis in tongue squamous cell carcinomas as an apoptosis inhibitor. Clin Cancer Res 15: 3998-4008, 2009.

[10] Yu J, Ryan DG, Getsios S, Oliveira-Fernandes M, Fatima A, Lavker RM: MicroRNA-184 antagonizes microRNA-205 to maintain SHIP2 levels in epithelia. Proc Natl Acad Sci U S A 105: 19300-19305, 2008.

[11] Dziunycz P, Iotzova-Weiss G, Eloranta JJ, Lauchli S, Hafner J, French LE, et al.: Squamous cell carcinoma of the skin shows a distinct microRNA profile modulated by UV radiation. J Invest Dermatol 130: 2686-2689, 2010.

[12] Sand M, Skrygan M, Sand D, Georgas D, Hahn S, Gambichler T, et al.: Expression of microRNAs in basal cell carcinoma. Br J Dermatol, 2012.

[13] Zhang JD, Biczok R, Ruschhaupt M: The ddCt Algorithm for the Analysis of Quantitative Real-Time PCR (qRT-PCR). 2011.

[14] Edgar R, Domrachev M, Lash AE: Gene Expression Omnibus: NCBI gene expression and hybridization array data repository. Nucleic Acids Res 30: 207-210, 2002.

[15] Sokal R, Michener C: A statistical method for evaluating systematic relationships. . University of Kansas Science Bulletin 38: 1409-1438, 1958.

[16] Quackenbush J: Computational analysis of microarray data. Nat Rev Genet 2: 418-427, 2001.

[17] Benjamini Y, Hochberg Y: Controlling the false discovery rate: a practical and powerful approach to multiple testing. J R Stat Soc Ser B 57: 289-300, 1995.

[18] Jiang Q, Wang Y, Hao Y, Juan L, Teng M, Zhang X, et al.: miR2Disease: a manually curated database for microRNA deregulation in human disease. Nucleic Acids Res 37: D98-104, 2009.

[19] Rowe DE, Carroll RJ, Day CL, Jr.: Prognostic factors for local recurrence, metastasis, and survival rates in squamous cell carcinoma of the skin, ear, and lip. Implications for treatment modality selection. J Am Acad Dermatol 26: 976-990, 1992.

[20] Marionnet C, Lalou C, Mollier K, Chazal M, Delestaing G, Compan D, et al.: Differential molecular profiling between skin carcinomas reveals four newly reported genes potentially implicated in squamous cell carcinoma development. Oncogene 22: 3500-3505, 2003.

[21] Feber A, Xi L, Luketich JD, Pennathur A, Landreneau RJ, Wu M, et al.: MicroRNA expression profiles of esophageal cancer. J Thorac Cardiovasc Surg 135: 255-260; discussion 260, 2008.

[22] Lu J, Getz G, Miska EA, Alvarez-Saavedra E, Lamb J, Peck D, et al.: MicroRNA expression profiles classify human cancers. Nature 435: 834-838, 2005.

[23] Hiyoshi Y, Kamohara H, Karashima R, Sato N, Imamura Y, Nagai Y, et al.: MicroRNA-21 regulates the proliferation and invasion in esophageal squamous cell carcinoma. Clin Cancer Res 15: 1915-1922, 2009.

[24] Liu M, Wu H, Liu T, Li Y, Wang F, Wan H, et al.: Regulation of the cell cycle gene, BTG2, by miR-21 in human laryngeal carcinoma. Cell Res 19: 828-837, 2009.

[25] Yu T, Wang XY, Gong RG, Li A, Yang S, Cao YT, et al.: The expression profile of microRNAs in a model of 7,12-dimethyl-benz[a]anthrance-induced oral carcinogenesis in Syrian hamster. J Exp Clin Cancer Res 28: 64, 2009.

[26] Gabriely G, Wurdinger T, Kesari S, Esau CC, Burchard J, Linsley PS, et al.: MicroRNA 21 promotes glioma invasion by targeting matrix metalloproteinase regulators. Mol Cell Biol 28: 5369-5380, 2008.

[27] Hufbauer M, Lazic D, Reinartz M, Akgul B, Pfister H, Weissenborn SJ: Skin tumor formation in human papillomavirus 8 transgenic mice is associated with a deregulation of oncogenic miRNAs and their tumor suppressive targets. J Dermatol Sci 64: 7-15, 2011.

[28] Zhu S, Si ML, Wu H, Mo YY: MicroRNA-21 targets the tumor suppressor gene tropomyosin 1 (TPM1). J Biol Chem 282: 14328-14336, 2007.

[29] Pesta M, Kulda V, Topolcan O, Safranek J, Vrzalova J, Cerny R, et al.: Significance of methylation status and the expression of RECK mRNA in lung tissue of patients with NSCLC. Anticancer Res 29: 4535-4539, 2009.

[30] Kettunen E, Anttila S, Seppanen JK, Karjalainen A, Edgren H, Lindstrom I, et al.: Differentially expressed genes in nonsmall cell lung cancer: expression profiling of cancer-related genes in squamous cell lung cancer. Cancer Genet Cytogenet 149: 98-106, 2004.

[31] Olive V, Jiang I, He L: mir-17-92, a cluster of miRNAs in the midst of the cancer network. Int J Biochem Cell Biol 42: 1348-1354, 2010.

[32] Uziel T, Karginov FV, Xie S, Parker JS, Wang YD, Gajjar A, et al.: The miR-17~92 cluster collaborates with the Sonic Hedgehog pathway in medulloblastoma. Proc Natl Acad Sci U S A 106: 2812-2817, 2009.

[33] Li C, Chi S, Xie J: Hedgehog signaling in skin cancers. Cell Signal 23: 1235-1243, 2011.

[34] Foekens JA, Sieuwerts AM, Smid M, Look MP, de Weerd V, Boersma AW, et al.: Four miRNAs associated with aggressiveness of lymph node-negative, estrogen receptor-positive human breast cancer. Proc Natl Acad Sci U S A 105: 13021-13026, 2008.

[35] Kim JH, Chang JH, Yoon JH, Lee JG, Bae JH, Kim KS: 15-Lipoxygenase-1 induced by interleukin-4 mediates apoptosis in oral cavity cancer cells. Oral Oncol 42: 825-830, 2006.

[36] Yeung ML, Yasunaga J, Bennasser Y, Dusetti N, Harris D, Ahmad N, et al.: Roles for microRNAs, miR-93 and miR-130b, and tumor protein 53-induced nuclear protein 1 tumor suppressor in cell growth dysregulation by human T-cell lymphotrophic virus 1. Cancer Res 68: 8976-8985, 2008.

[37] Wong TS, Liu XB, Chung-Wai Ho A, Po-Wing Yuen A, Wai-Man Ng R, Ignace Wei W: Identification of pyruvate kinase type M2 as potential oncoprotein in squamous cell carcinoma of tongue through microRNA profiling. Int J Cancer 123: 251-257, 2008.

[38] Su H, Yang JR, Xu T, Huang J, Xu L, Yuan Y, et al.: MicroRNA-101, down-regulated in hepatocellular carcinoma, promotes apoptosis and suppresses tumorigenicity. Cancer Res 69: 1135-1142, 2009.

[39] Nagata M, Wada K, Nakajima A, Nakajima N, Kusayama M, Masuda T, et al.: Role of myeloid cell leukemia-1 in cell growth of squamous cell carcinoma. J Pharmacol Sci 110: 344-353, 2009.

[40] Kozaki K, Imoto I, Mogi S, Omura K, Inazawa J: Exploration of tumor-suppressive microRNAs silenced by DNA hypermethylation in oral cancer. Cancer Res 68: 2094-2105, 2008.

[41] Lee Y, Yang X, Huang Y, Fan H, Zhang Q, Wu Y, et al.: Network modeling identifies molecular functions targeted by miR-204 to suppress head and neck tumor metastasis. PLoS Comput Biol 6: e1000730, 2010.

[42] Munding JB, Adai AT, Maghnouj A, Urbanik A, Zollner H, Liffers ST, et al.: Global microRNA expression profiling of microdissected tissues identifies miR-135b as a novel biomarker for pancreatic ductal adenocarcinoma. Int J Cancer 131: E86-95, 2012.

[43] Matsuyama H, Suzuki HI, Nishimori H, Noguchi M, Yao T, Komatsu N, et al.: miR-135b mediates NPM-ALK-driven oncogenicity and renders IL-17-producing immunophenotype to anaplastic large cell lymphoma. Blood 118: 6881-6892, 2011.

[44] Ghosh G, Subramanian IV, Adhikari N, Zhang X, Joshi HP, Basi D, et al.: Hypoxia-induced microRNA-424 expression in human endothelial cells regulates HIF-alpha isoforms and promotes angiogenesis. J Clin Invest 120: 4141-4154, 2010.

[45] Chamorro-Jorganes A, Araldi E, Penalva LO, Sandhu D, Fernandez-Hernando C, Suarez Y: MicroRNA-16 and microRNA-424 regulate cell-autonomous angiogenic functions in endothelial cells via targeting vascular endothelial growth factor receptor-2 and fibroblast growth factor receptor-1. Arterioscler Thromb Vasc Biol 31: 2595-2606, 2011.

[46] Lu J, He ML, Wang L, Chen Y, Liu X, Dong Q, et al.: MiR-26a inhibits cell growth and tumorigenesis of nasopharyngeal carcinoma through repression of EZH2. Cancer Res 71: 225-233, 2011.

[47] Sander S, Bullinger L, Klapproth K, Fiedler K, Kestler HA, Barth TF, et al.: MYC stimulates EZH2 expression by repression of its negative regulator miR-26a. Blood 112: 4202-4212, 2008.

[48] Kumarswamy R, Mudduluru G, Ceppi P, Muppala S, Kozlowski M, Niklinski J, et al.: MicroRNA-30a inhibits epithelial-to-mesenchymal transition by targeting Snai1 and is downregulated in non-small cell lung cancer. Int J Cancer 130: 2044-2053, 2012.

[49] Baraniskin A, Birkenkamp-Demtroder K, Maghnouj A, Zollner H, Munding J, Klein-Scory S, et al.: MiR-30a-5p suppresses tumor growth in colon carcinoma by targeting DTL. Carcinogenesis 33: 732-739, 2012.

[50] Jude JA, Dileepan M, Subramanian S, Solway J, Panettieri RA, Jr., Walseth TF, et al.: miR-140-3p regulation of TNF-alpha-induced CD38 expression in human airway smooth muscle cells. Am J Physiol Lung Cell Mol Physiol 303: L460-468, 2012.

[51] Kano M, Seki N, Kikkawa N, Fujimura L, Hoshino I, Akutsu Y, et al.: miR-145, miR-133a and miR-133b: Tumor-suppressive miRNAs target FSCN1 in esophageal squamous cell carcinoma. Int J Cancer 127: 2804-2814, 2010.

[52] Knezevic I, Patel A, Sundaresan NR, Gupta MP, Solaro RJ, Nagalingam RS, et al.: A novel cardiomyocyte-enriched microRNA, miR-378, targets insulin-like growth factor 1 receptor: implications in postnatal cardiac remodeling and cell survival. J Biol Chem 287: 12913-12926, 2012.

[53] Fang J, Song XW, Tian J, Chen HY, Li DF, Wang JF, et al.: Overexpression of microRNA-378 attenuates ischemia-induced apoptosis by inhibiting caspase-3 expression in cardiac myocytes. Apoptosis 17: 410-423, 2012.

9 Paper 5: The miRNA machinery in primary cutaneous malignant melanoma, cutaneous malignant melanoma metastases and benign melanocytic nevi*

9.1 Introduction

MicroRNAs (miRNAs) are 17- to 21-nucleotide (nt) short RNAs and represent a relatively new class of molecules that regulate gene expression on a post-transcriptional level by binding to target mRNA, resulting in mRNA degradation or the inhibition of mRNA translation (Bartel, 2004, Sand, et al., 2009). It has been estimated that miRNAs play a pivotal role in post-transcriptional gene regulation in up to 30-60% of all human genes while some authors even speculate that every gene in the genome, regardless if it´s coding or not, can be regulated by miRNAs (Bonazzi, et al., 2011, Friedman, et al., 2009, Lewis, et al., 2005). miRNA maturation begins in the nucleus, where the primary-miRNA (pri-miRNA) transcript is transcribed by RNA polymerase II (Lee, et al., 2002). The intranuclear RNase III endonuclease Drosha, together with DiGeorge syndrome critical region gene 8 (DGCR8 or Pasha), build the microprocessor complex, which cleaves the pri-miRNA transcript within the nucleus into several precursor miRNAs (pre-miRNAs) (Gregory, et al., 2004). Drosha is the catalytic subunit of the pri-miRNA processing intranuclear microprocessor complex, while DGCR8 stabilizes Drosha and recognizes the RNA substrate (Han, et al., 2004, Landthaler, et al., 2004). The 70- to 90-nt-long pre-miRNAs are then transported to the cytoplasm by the miRNA nuclear export receptor RAN GTPase Exportin-5 (Exp5) and are processed by Dicer, another RNase III enzyme (Kim, 2004). The product is a mature miRNA strand that can be incorporated into the 200- to 500-kDa multiprotein miRNA effector complex that possesses endonuclease activity and is called the RNA-induced silencing complex (RISC). Dicer is not only a cytosolic miRNA maturing RNase III enzyme; it is also a part of the RISC (Gregory, et al.,

---

* Co-authors: Marina Skrygan, Ph.D., Dimitrios Georgas, M.D., Daniel Sand, M.D., Thilo Gambichler, M.D., Peter Altmeyer, M.D., Falk G. Bechara, M.D.

2005). The miRNA / RISC complex anneals to the target mRNA in the so called "seed region" on the miRNA nts 2-7; in the event of nearly complete complementarity, endonucleolytic cleavage of the target mRNA occurs, resulting in a cessation of translation (Dalmay, 2008). In the event of limited complementarity, however, translation is only suppressed (Reinhart, et al., 2000). Besides the miRNA processing enzyme Dicer, the components described below have also been determined to be part of the RISC.

Argonaute-1 (AGO1, eukaryotic translation initiation factor 2C.1, EIF2C1) and argonaute-2 (AGO2, eukaryotic translation initiation factor 2C.2, EIF2C2) are the actual mRNA slicing catalytic subunits of the RISC, which catalyze message degradation (Faehnle and Joshua-Tor, 2007). The double-stranded RNA binding proteins (dsRBP) Dicer-substrate complex stabilizing methyltransferase TAR HIV-1 RNA binding protein 1 (TARBP1) and RISC-loading complex subunit TAR HIV-1 RNA binding protein 2 (TARBP2) are also well-described RISC components. Protein activator of protein kinase R (PACT) is another dsRBP and is part of the RISC (Lee, et al., 2006). Metadherin (MTDH), also known as protein LYRIC or astrocyte elevated gene-1 protein (AEG-1), is an oncoprotein that is reported to be overexpressed in a variety of cancers, including primary cutaneous malignant melanoma (Kim, et al., 2011). It has been described as a part of the RISC and is additionally known to be a significant positive activator of the transcription factor nuclear factor-kappaB (NF-kappaB), which controls the expression of multiple genes involved in tumor progression and metastasis (Emdad, et al., 2006, Yoo, et al., 2011). Another component of the RISC is staphylococcal nuclease and tudor domain containing 1 (SND1) (Caudy, et al., 2003). SND1 is a multifunctional regulator protein of gene expression that is cleaved by caspase-3 during apoptosis. It is a miRNAse that has been shown to play multiple roles in transcriptional regulation, RNA splicing and RNA interference (Li, et al., 2008).

Previously, a few studies have indicated possible perturbations in the miRNA machinery of primary cutaneous malignant melanoma (Ma, et al., 2011, Sand, et al., 2011a). Therefore, this study was initiated to compare the mRNA expression levels of well-described components of miRNA maturation (Dicer and the microprocessor complex), transport (Exp5) and effect (the RISC) in primary cutaneous malignant melanoma (PCMM), cutaneous malignant melanoma metastases (CMMM) and benign melanocytic nevi (BMN).

9.2 Materials and Methods

This study was approved by the Ethical Review Board of the Ruhr-University Bochum, Germany (registration number: 3265-08, ClinicalTrials.gov Identifier: NCT01444560) and originates from a section of dermatologic surgery at an academic hospital of the Ruhr-University Bochum (Germany). It was conducted within the framework of the declaration of Helsinki. Informed consents were signed by all study subjects.

9.2.1 Subjects

Seven patients (1 female, 6 males; median age: 75 years) with PCMM (3 SSM, 1 ALM, 3 NM), six patients with CMMM (2 females, 4 males; median age: 67 years) and seven patients with BMN (4 females, 3 males; median age: 16 years) that served as controls were enrolled in this study (see table 9-1 for details). Skin tumors were excised with scalpels under local anesthesia. Specimens were obtained with a 4-mm punch biopsy from the tumor center and were immediately stored in RNAlater (Qiagen, Hilden, Germany) and kept at -80 °C until RNA isolation.

9.2.2 RNA isolation and TaqMan real-time reverse transcription polymerase chain reaction (RT-PCR)

Total cellular RNA was isolated from tissue samples using the miRNeasy Mini Kit (Qiagen, Chatsworth, CA, USA) following the manufacturer's protocol. An aliquot of each of the isolated total RNA samples was used to determine total RNA concentrations and A260/280 ratios on a NanoDrop ND-1000 spectrophotometer (Peqlab, Erlangen, Germany). Additionally, all samples were analyzed using RNA 6000 Nano LabChip Kits (Agilent Technologies) on a 2100 Bioanalyzer (Agilent Technolo-gies) to determine their RNA integrity numbers (RIN) on a scale from 1 –

10. According to the recommendations of Fleige and Pfaffl, we defined a minimum RIN > 5 to be suitable for further consideration by TaqMan RT-PCR analysis (Fleige and Pfaffl, 2006). The High-Capacity cDNA Reverse Transcription Kit (Applied Biosystems) was used for reverse transcription of total RNA into single-stranded cDNA with the aid of random hexamer primers according to the manufacturer's instructions. One microgram of total RNA was reverse transcribed in a total volume of 50 µl. Inventoried and made-to-order TaqMan Gene expression assays (Applied Biosystems, Darmstadt, Germany) were used for RNA expression analysis of the following target genes: Dicer (TaqMan Assay ID Hs00229023_m1), Drosha (Hs00203008_m1), Exp5 (Hs00382453_m1), DGCR8 (Hs00377897_m1), PACT (Hs00269379_m1), argonaute-1 (Hs00201864_m1), argonaute-2 (Hs01085579_m1), TARBP1 (Hs0019 4596_m1), TARBP2 (Hs00366328_m1), MTDH (Hs00757841_m1) and SND1 (Hs00205182_m1). To improve the accuracy of determining expression levels, the three reference genes β-glucuronidase (GUSB, Hs00939627_m1), hypoxanthine phosphoribosyltransferase (HPRT, Hs01003267_m1) and ribosomal protein L38 (RPL38, Hs01019602_g1) were chosen according to de Kok et al. (de Kok, et al., 2005). The qPCR analysis was performed in technical triplicates according to the manufacturer's instructions using the TaqMan Universal MasterMix II (Applied Biosystems, Darmstadt, Germany) with uracil-N-glycosylase (UNG) and 20 ng cDNA in a final reaction volume of 10 µl. The reaction mix was transferred into 384-well plates; after sealing, the plates were run on an AB7900HT instrument (Applied Biosystems, Darmstadt, Germany). The following temperature profile was used: 50°C / 2:00 min – 95°C / 10:00 min – [95°C / 0:15 min – 60°C / 1:00 min] x 40 cycles. The software Sequence Detection Systems *SDS 2.4* (Applied Biosystems, Darmstadt, Germany) was employed for instrument control, data acquisition and raw data analysis. The plates were run in *Relative Quantification* ($\Delta\Delta C_t$) mode. For qRT-PCR data analysis, the $\Delta\Delta C_t$ method was applied as previously described by Zhang et al. (Zhang, et al., 2011). Bioconductor package $\Delta\Delta C_t$ (v1.5.0) was implemented for the advanced calculation of relative expression levels in this study. Briefly, the expression levels of target RNAs were standardized to the

expression levels of three reference RNAs and related to the expression levels of target and reference RNAs in a calibrator sample. This analysis was performed using the sample from patient 1 as the calibrator sample and the means of the reference genes GUSB, HPRT and RPL38.

9.2.3   Statistical analyses

Data analysis was performed using Med-Calc software version 11.6.0.0 (Mariakerke, Belgium). The null hypothesis was based on the assumption that there are no differences in Dicer, Drosha, Exp-5, DGCR8, PACT, argonaute-1, argonaute-2, TARBP1, TARBP2, MTDH and SND-1 expression levels between the three groups (PCMM, CMMM and BMN) in this study. The analysis of data distribution was assessed by the Kolmogorov-Smirnov test. Prior to the ANOVA test, Levene's test for equality of variances was performed. When the Levene's test was significant (as for TARBP2 ($P<0.05$)), the Kruskal-Wallis test was performed.

When the Levene's test was not significant ($P>0.05$), one-way ANOVA for three independent samples was used for inter-arm comparisons. Subsequently, the Student-Newman-Keuls or the Conover test for pairwise comparisons was used to determine which groups showed significantly different expression levels. Additionally, the Pearson or Spearman correlation coefficients (r) were analyzed. All results were expressed as means ± standard deviations (SD) or medians and range (TARBP2), with statistical significance set at 5% (two-sided).

Tab. 9-1: A= absent, ALM= acral lentiginous melanoma, BMN=benign melanocytic nevi, CL=Clark level, CMMM= cutaneous malignant melanoma metastases, n.a.= not available, NMM= nodular malignant melanoma, P= present, PCMM= primary cutaneous malignant melanoma, RIN= RNA integrity number, SSM= superficial spreading melanoma, TT= tumor thickness, mm=millimeters.

Patient Number	Sex	Age	Localization	Histology	Ulcer-ation	Mitoses	RNA conc. (ng/µl)	A260/280 ratio	RIN
PCMM1	f	84	foot	ALM, TT 3.2 mm, pT3	n.a.	n.a.	184.82	2.09	9.2
PCMM2	m	73	epigastrium	NMM, TT 3.8 mm, CL IV, pT3b	P	$<1\,/mm^2$	444.22	1.92	9.2
PCMM3	m	76	lower leg	SSM, TT 3.2 mm, CL IV, pT3a	A	$>1\,/mm^2$	210.71	2.06	8.0
PCMM4	m	84	back	SSM, TT 3.8 mm, CL IV, pT3a	A	$>1\,/mm^2$	331.66	2.07	7.5
PCMM5	m	47	buttock	SSM, TT 2.1 mm, CL IV, pT3b	P	$>1\,/mm^2$	637.64	2.08	7.8
PCMM6	m	86	lower leg	NMM, TT 1.4 mm, CL IV, pT2b	P	n.a.	137.29	2.05	9.1
PCMM7	m	79	popliteal fossa	NMM, TT 1.5 mm, CL IV, pT2a	A	n.a.	96.64	2.07	8.9

Tab. 9-1: (Continued)

Patient Number	Sex	Age	Localization	Histology	Ulcer-ation	Mitoses	RNA conc. (ng/µl)	A260/280 ratio	RIN
CMMM-1	f	70	thigh	CMMM			128.78	2.04	9.0
CMMM-2	m	76	thigh	CMMM			641.07	2.11	7.2
CMMM-3	f	84	lower leg	CMMM			628.95	2.08	5.7
CMMM-4	m	52	shoulder	CMMM			2446.10	2.08	5.4
CMMM-5	m	69	iliac crest	CMMM			1518.82	2.03	6.9
CMMM-6	m	53	back	CMMM			1139.23	2.09	5.7
BMN-1	f	13	back of neck	BMN			458.64	2.08	5.1
BMN-2	f	13	flank	BMN			150.47	2.11	8.9
BMN-3	m	23	lower leg	BMN			69.38	2.02	8.5
BMN-4	m	9	upper arm	BMN			114.29	2.03	8.6
BMN-5	f	12	abdomen	BMN			117.55	2.06	8.6
BMN-6	m	25	shoulder	BMN			298.76	2.08	9.1
BMN-7	f	18	back of neck	BMN			62.33	2.06	7.7

Fig. 9-1:   Multiple-comparison Box-and-Whisker plots showing argonaute-1 (Fig 9-1a), argonaute-2 (Fig 9-1b), TARBP2 (Fig 9-1c), SND1 (Fig 9-1d), Dicer (Fig 9-1e), Drosha (Fig 9-1f), DGCR8 (Fig 9-1g), Exp5 (Fig 9-1h), PACT (Fig 9-1i), TARBP1 (Fig 9-1j) and MTDH (Fig 9-1k) mRNA expression levels relative to the mRNA expression levels for the reference genes GUSB, HPRT and RPL38 in primary cutaneous malignant melanoma (PCMM), cutaneous malignant melanoma metastases (CMMM) and benign melanocytic nevi (BMN).

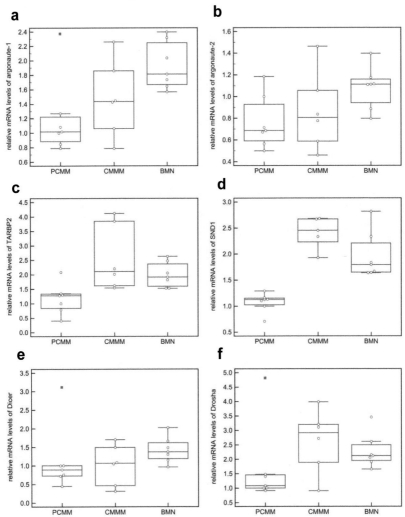

Fig. 9-1:   (Continued)

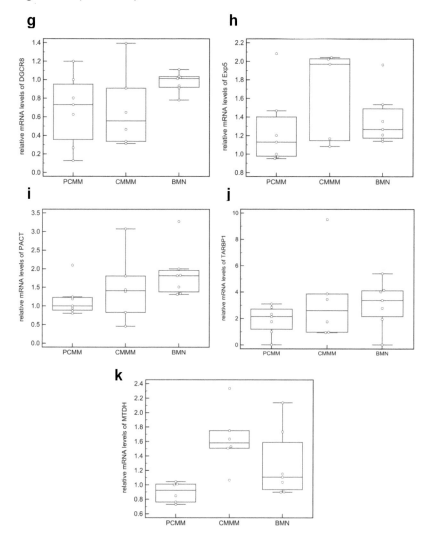

9.3   Results

The expression levels of argonaute-1 were significantly higher in BMN compared to PCMM (*p*<0.05; Figure 9-1a). The expression levels of argonaute-2 were not significantly different between groups (*p*>0.05;

Figure 9-1b). TARBP2 expression levels were significantly higher in BMN compared to PCMM and in CMMM compared to PCMM ($p<0.05$; Figure 9-1c). SND1 expression levels were significantly higher in BMN compared to PCMM and in CMMM compared to PCMM and BMN ($p<0.05$; Figure 9-1d). Dicer, Drosha, DGCR8, Exp5, PACT, TARBP1 and MTDH expression levels showed no significant differences within the three groups ($p>0.05$; Figure 9-1e–k). Details of the quantitative real-time PCR data are given in table 9-2. Analyses of the correlations of each target gene among the others between groups were performed. The following pairs with very significant degrees of correlation ($p<0.01$) were identified for PCMM: Dicer/Drosha, Dicer/argonaute-1, Dicer/PACT, Dicer/MTDH, Drosha/argonaute-1, Drosha/PACT, Drosha/MTDH, argo-naute-1/PACT, argonaute-1/MTDH and PACT/MTDH. The correlation pair ($p<0.01$) identified for CMMM was argonaute-1/PACT. The correlation pairs ($p<.01$) for BMN were Dicer/Exp5, Dicer/argonaute-1, Dicer/MTDH, Dicer/SND1, Exp5/argonaute-1, Exp5/MTDH, Exp5/SND1, argonaute-1/MTDH and MTDH/SND1. For details, see table 9-3.

9.4   Discussion

Disruptions of the miRNA machinery have previously been linked to a variety of different cancers (Gartel and Kandel, 2006). While investigating the role of miRNA in PCMM, studies have recently focused on reporting differences in miRNA expression profiles of cutaneous malignant melanoma cells compared to benign melanocytes (Mueller, et al., 2009). Additionally, a few functional studies have highlighted the roles of some specific miRNAs in cutaneous melanoma (Bonazzi, Stark and Hayward, 2011, Glud, et al., 2011, Howell, et al., 2010, Mueller, Rehli and Bosserhoff, 2009). The expression of the miRNA machinery itself, which consists of extra- and intranuclear miRNA maturation components (Dicer, Drosha and microprocessor complex component DGCR8), the nuclear pre-miRNA transport receptor (Exportin-5 or Exp5) and the extracellular miRNA effector RISC (Dicer, argonaute-1, argonaute-2, TARBP1, TARBP2, PACT, MTDH and SND1), have not been systematically investigated in PCMM. A dysregulation of the miRNA-maturing enzyme Dicer and other RISC components has been described for epithelial skin cancers on the mRNA level and for PCMM on the mRNA and protein levels (Ma, Swede, Cassarino, Fleming, Fire and Dadras, 2011, Sand, Gambichler, Sand, Altmeyer, Stuecker and Bechara, 2011a, Sand, et al., 2010, Sand, et al., 2011b). Further, a pilot study revealed a significant increase in Dicer expression for formalin-fixed PCMM by immunohistochemistry compared to benign melanocytic nevi, which was recently confirmed in another larger study (Ma, Swede, Cassarino, Fleming, Fire and Dadras, 2011, Sand, Gambichler, Sand, Altmeyer, Stuecker and Bechara, 2011a). Further, a bioinformatic pooled analysis based on publicly available gene expression profiling studies previously performed on whole-genome oligo-microarray platforms presumed an up-regulation of Dicer and DGRC8 from a common melanocytic nevus to invasive cutaneous melanoma. A down-regulation of Drosha was described for melanoma in situ to invasive melanoma and for Exp5 in metastatic melanoma compared to normal skin (Riker, et al., 2008, Scatolini, et al., 2010). However, all of these latter preliminary microarray screening results have not yet been validated.

This study does not confirm these preliminary findings in our collective of patients, demonstrating that not all of the major components of the miRNA machinery are significantly dysregulated in PCMM or CMMM compared to BMN. Although based on a limited number of patients, our data still shows on a significant level ($p<0.05$) that three components of the miRNA machinery (argonaute-1, TARBP2 and SND1), which are all part of the miRNA effector RISC, are dysregulated. All dysregulated targets (argonaute-1, TARBP2 and SND1) are components of the RISC and were significantly under-expressed ($p<0.05$) in PCMM compared to BMN. Nevertheless the sizes of the samples in this study are small and the results should be further validated in a larger study.

Tab. 9-2: Quantitative TaqMan real-time RT-PCR data showing Dicer, Drosha, DGCR8, Exp5, argonaute-1, argonaute-2, PACT, TARBP1, TARBP2, MTDH and SND1 (mean ± SD) expression levels from primary cutaneous malignant melanoma (PCMM, n = 7), cutaneous malignant melanoma metastases (CMMM, n = 6) and benign melanocytic nevi (BMN, n = 7), relative to expression levels of reference genes β-glucuronidase, HPRT and RPL38. HPRT= hypoxanthine ribosyltransferase, RPL38 = human ribosomal protein R38 (reference genes). All data are relative expression levels. * = Statistically significant difference.

Parameter	PCMM (a)	CMMM (b)	BMN (c)
Dicer	1.13 ± 0.9	1.02 ± 0.55	1.42 ± 0.35
Drosha	1.67 ± 1.4	2.63 ± 1.09	2.28 ± 0.6
DGCR8	0.68 ± 0.38	0.68 ± 0.41	0.97 ± 0.11
Exp5	1.26 ± 0.41	2.17 ± 1.33	1.38 ± 0.29
argonaute-1	1.2 ± 0.54 a versus c*	1.47 ± 0.53	1.93 ± 0.33
argonaute-2	0.76 ± 0.25	0.86 ± 0.36	1.08 ± 0.19
PACT	1.16 ± 0.44	1.5 ± 0.91	1.87 ± 0.67
TARBP1	1.89 ± 1.08	3.41 ± 3.23	3.1 ± 1.75
TARBP2	1.28 (0.40 – 2.08) a versus b* a versus c*	2.11 (2.56 – 4.19)	1.91 (1.52 – 2.63)
MTDH	1.84 ± 2.5	1.64 ± 0.41	1.28 ± 0.47
SND1	1.07 ± 0.18 a versus b* a versus c*	2.81 ± 1	1.96 ± 0.45

Although Holst et al. were able to show that the actual miRNA expression pattern in normal human skin is reproducible in different ages and body locations this is not necessarily the case for the miRNA machinery components investigated in the present study (Holst, et al., 2010). It is therefore important to keep in mind the age differences between the BMN group (median age:16 years) and the melanoma group (PCMM group median age:75 years, CMMM group median age:67 years) as the age might have an influence.

Correlation analysis shows that in the PCMM group, we were able to identify 10 pairs of target genes, 7 of the pairs consisting exclusively of RISC members and 3 pairs consisting of one RISC member and Drosha, all with very significant degrees of correlation ($p<0.01$). In CMMM, we found only one very significant ($p<0.01$) correlation pair. In BMN, we identified 9 very significant ($p<0.01$) correlation pairs, 4 of which involved Exp5 and one member of the RISC. It remains unclear why the miRNA nuclear export receptor Exp5 is often noticeably co-expressed in correlation with other members of the miRNA machinery on a very significant level only in BMN ($p<0.01$). One could speculate that during melanoma formation or metastasis, the expression of Exp5 uncouples from the other members of miRNA machinery.

Whether the observed dysregulation of the previously described components of the miRNA machinery in this pilot study have any actual pathological roles within melanoma formation or whether the significant findings are a consequence of tumor formation cannot be answered based on our data. Nevertheless, we expect that larger studies will be able to enlighten the possible role of the miRNA machinery in PCMM or in CMMM.

Tab. 9-3: Pearson correlation coefficient (r), P-value (p). The correlation is significant (two-sided) with $p<0.05$ (*); the correlation is very significant (two-sided) with $p<0.01$ (**). Primary cutaneous malignant melanoma (PCMM), cutaneous malignant melanoma metastases (CMMM), benign melanocytic nevi (BMN).

		Dicer	Drosha	DGCR8	EXP5	argonaute-1	argonaute-2
Dicer	PCMM r =		,986 (**)	-,621	,256	,980 (**)	-,339
	PCMM p =		,000	,136	,580	,000	,457
	CMMM r =		-,160	-,673	-,578	-,767	-,316
	CMMM p =		,762	,143	,229	,075	,542
	BMN r =		,517	,699	,941 (**)	,948 (**)	,684
	BMN p =		,235	,080	,002	,001	,090
Drosha	PCMM r =	,986 (**)		-,651	,292	,984 (**)	-,405
	PCMM p =	,000		,113	,524	,000	,367
	CMMM r =	-,160		,240	-,007	,441	,043
	CMMM p =	,762		,646	,990	,381	,935
	BMN r =	,517		,285	,566	,709	,584
	BMN p =	,235		,536	,185	,074	,168
DGCR8	PCMM r =	-,621	-,651		,356	-,663	,798 (*)
	PCMM p =	,136	,113		,433	,105	,031
	CMMM r =	-,673	,240		,839 (*)	,581	,760
	CMMM p =	,143	,646		,037	,227	,080
	BMN r =	,699	,285		,503	,726	,799 (*)
	BMN p =	,080	,536		,250	,065	,031

Tab. 9-3:   (Continued)

		PACT	TARBP1	TARBP2	MTDH	SND1
Dicer	PCMM r =	,946 (**)	,510	-,666	,984 (**)	,011
	PCMM p =	,001	,242	,102	,000	,981
	CMMM r =	-,748	,317	-,177	-,813 (*)	,076
	CMMM p =	,087	,540	,738	,049	,887
	BMN r =	,741	,249	,654	,942 (**)	,888 (**)
	BMN p =	,057	,590	,111	,001	,008
Drosha	PCMM r =	,945 (**)	,558	-,624	,992 (**)	,043
	PCMM p =	,001	,193	,134	,000	,927
	CMMM r =	,363	,294	,367	,041	-,875 (*)
	CMMM p =	,479	,572	,475	,939	,022
	BMN r =	,000	,083	,332	,700	,672
	BMN p =	1,000	,860	,467	,080	,098
DGCR8	PCMM r =	-,675	-,600	,844 (*)	-,632	,333
	PCMM p =	,096	,154	,017	,128	,465
	CMMM r =	,470	,288	,340	,731	-,121
	CMMM p =	,347	,580	,509	,099	,819
	BMN r =	,372	-,149	,460	,507	,350
	BMN p =	,412	,749	,298	,245	,441

Tab. 9-3: (Continued)

		Dicer	Drosha	DGCR8	EXP5	argonaute-1	argonaute-2
EXP5	PCMM r =	,256	,292	,356		,247	,535
	PCMM p =	,580	,524	,433		,593	,216
	CMMM r =	-,578	-,007	,839 (*)		,413	,880 (*)
	CMMM p =	,229	,990	,037		,415	,021
	BMN r =	,941 (**)	,566	,503		,912 (**)	,478
	BMN p =	,002	,185	,250		,004	,278
argonaute-1	PCMM r =	,980 (**)	,984 (**)	-,663	,247		-,362
	PCMM p =	,000	,000	,105	,593		,425
	CMMM r =	-,767	,441	,581	,413		,459
	CMMM p =	,075	,381	,227	,415		,360
	BMN r =	,948 (**)	,709	,726	,912 (**)		,768 (*)
	BMN p =	,001	,074	,065	,004		,044
argonaute-2	PCMM r =	-,339	-,405	,798 (*)	,535	-,362	
	PCMM p =	,457	,367	,031	,216	,425	
	CMMM r =	-,316	,043	,760	,880 (*)	,459	
	CMMM p =	,542	,935	,080	,021	,360	
	BMN r =	,684	,584	,799 (*)	,478	,768 (*)	
	BMN p =	,090	,168	,031	,278	,044	

Tab. 9-3: (Continued)

		PACT	TARBP1	TARBP2	MTDH	SND1
EXP5	PCMM r =	,130	,250	,539	,248	,417
	PCMM p =	,781	,589	,211	,592	,352
	CMMM r =	,252	-,127	-,201	,903(*)	,096
	CMMM p =	,630	,811	,702	,014	,857
	BMN r =	,788 (*)	,181	,744	,978 (**)	,953 (**)
	BMN p =	,035	,697	,055	,000	,001
argonaute-1	PCMM r =	,970 (**)	,526	-,669	,965 (**)	-,114
	PCMM p =	,000	,225	,100	,000	,808
	CMMM r =	,976 (**)	-,035	,436	,550	-,601
	CMMM p =	,001	,947	,388	,258	,207
	BMN r =	,548	,063	,704	,945 (**)	,859 (*)
	BMN p =	,203	,893	,078	,001	,013
argonaute-2	PCMM r =	-,454	-,215	,668	-,434	-,027
	PCMM p =	,306	,644	,101	,330	,954
	CMMM r =	,301	,141	-,025	,654	-,140
	CMMM p =	,562	,789	,963	,159	,791
	BMN r =	,110	,161	,218	,591	,479
	BMN p =	,814	,730	,639	,163	,276

Tab. 9-3: (Continued)

		Dicer	Drosha	DGCR8	EXP5	argonaute-1	argonaute-2
PACT	PCMM r =	,946 (**)	,945 (**)	-,675	,130	,970 (**)	-,454
	PCMM p =	,001	,001	,096	,781	,000	,306
	CMMM r =	-,748	,363	,470	,252	,976 (**)	,301
	CMMM p =	,087	,479	,347	,630	,001	,562
	BMN r =	,741	,000	,372	,788(*)	,548	,110
	BMN p =	,057	1,000	,412	,035	,203	,814
TARBP1	PCMM r =	,510	,558	-,600	,250	,526	-,215
	PCMM p =	,242	,193	,154	,589	,225	,644
	CMMM r =	,317	,294	,288	-,127	-,035	,141
	CMMM p =	,540	,572	,580	,811	,947	,789
	BMN r =	,249	,083	-,149	,181	,063	,161
	BMN p =	,590	,860	,749	,697	,893	,730
TARBP2	PCMM r =	-,666	-,624	,844 (*)	,539	-,669	,668
	PCMM p =	,102	,134	,017	,211	,100	,101
	CMMM r =	-,177	,367	,340	-,201	,436	-,025
	CMMM p =	,738	,475	,509	,702	,388	,963
	BMN r =	,654	,332	,460	,744	,704	,218
	BMN p =	,111	,467	,298	,055	,078	,639

Tab. 9-3: (Continued)

		PACT	TARBP1	TARBP2	MTDH	SND1
PACT	PCMM r=		,342	-,717	,931 (**)	-,101
	PCMM p=		,452	,070	,002	,829
	CMMM r=		-,029	,521	,426	-,556
	CMMM p=		,956	,289	,400	,252
	BMN r=		,307	,525	,675	,700
	BMN p=		,504	,227	,096	,080
TARBP1	PCMM r=	,342		-,310	,520	-,180
	PCMM p=	,452		,498	,231	,699
	CMMM r=	-,029		,762	-,437	-,301
	CMMM p=	,956		,078	,386	,561
	BMN r=	,307		-,478	,254	,406
	BMN p=	,504		,278	,582	,366
TARBP2	PCMM r=	-,717	-,310		-,643	,410
	PCMM p=	,070	,498		,119	,361
	CMMM r=	,521	,762		-,267	-,447
	CMMM p=	,289	,078		,609	,374
	BMN r=	,525	-,478		,659	,548
	BMN p=	,227	,278		,107	,203

Tab. 9-3:   (Continued)

		Dicer	Drosha	DGCR8	EXP5	argonaute-1	argonaute-2
MTDH	PCMM r =	,984 (**)	,992 (**)	-,632	,248	,965 (**)	-,434
	PCMM p =	,000	,000	,128	,592	,000	,330
	CMMM r =	-,813 (*)	,041	,731	,903 (*)	,550	,654
	CMMM p =	,049	,939	,099	,014	,258	,159
	BMN r =	,942 (**)	,700	,507	,978 (**)	,945 (**)	,591
	BMN p =	,001	,080	,245	,000	,001	,163
SND1	PCMM r =	,011	,043	,333	,417	-,114	-,027
	PCMM p =	,981	,927	,465	,352	,808	,954
	CMMM r =	,076	-,875 (*)	-,121	,096	-,601	-,140
	CMMM p =	,887	,022	,819	,857	,207	,791
	BMN r =	,888 (**)	,672	,350	,953 (**)	,859 (*)	,479
	BMN p =	,008	,098	,441	,001	,013	,276

Tab. 9-3: (Continued)

		PACT	TARBP1	TARBP2	MTDH	SND1
MTDH	PCMM r =	,931 (**)	,520	-,643		,106
	PCMM p =	,002	,231	,119		,821
	CMMM r =	,426	-,437	-,267		,076
	CMMM p =	,400	,386	,609		,887
	BMN r =	,675	,254	,659		,977 (**)
	BMN p =	,096	,582	,107		,000
SND1	PCMM r =	-,101	-,180	,410	,106	
	PCMM p =	,829	,699	,361	,821	
	CMMM r =	-,556	-,301	-,447	,076	
	CMMM p =	,252	,561	,374	,887	
	BMN r =	,700	,406	,548	,977 (**)	
	BMN p =	,080	,366	,203	,000	

9.5   Conclusion

This study indicates that argonaute-1, TARBP2 and SND1 in PCMM and TARBP2 and SND1 in CMMM, all components of the RISC, are dysregulated within the miRNA machinery and should be further investigated in detail.

9.6   Acknowledgements

This work was generously supported in part by Fleur-Hiege-Stiftung-gegen-Hautkrebs, Hamburg, Germany. The authors are grateful to Dr. Cornelia Graf and Stefan Kotschote, M.S., for technical assistance.

9.7   References

Bartel DP (2004) MicroRNAs: genomics, biogenesis, mechanism, and function. Cell 116:281-297

Bonazzi VF, Stark MS, Hayward NK (2011) MicroRNA regulation of melanoma progression. Melanoma Res

Caudy AA, Ketting RF, Hammond SM, Denli AM, Bathoorn AM, Tops BB, Silva JM, Myers MM, Hannon GJ, Plasterk RH (2003) A micrococcal nuclease homologue in RNAi effector complexes. Nature 425:411-414

Dalmay T (2008) Identification of genes targeted by microRNAs. Biochem Soc Trans 36:1194-1196

de Kok JB, Roelofs RW, Giesendorf BA, Pennings JL, Waas ET, Feuth T, Swinkels DW, Span PN (2005) Normalization of gene expression measurements in tumor tissues: comparison of 13 endogenous control genes. Lab Invest 85:154-159

Emdad L, Sarkar D, Su ZZ, Randolph A, Boukerche H, Valerie K, Fisher PB (2006) Activation of the nuclear factor kappaB pathway by astrocyte elevated gene-1: implications for tumor progression and metastasis. Cancer Res 66:1509-1516

Faehnle CR, Joshua-Tor L (2007) Argonautes confront new small RNAs. Curr Opin Chem Biol 11:569-577

Fleige S, Pfaffl MW (2006) RNA integrity and the effect on the real-time qRT-PCR performance. Mol Aspects Med 27:126-139

Friedman RC, Farh KK, Burge CB, Bartel DP (2009) Most mammalian mRNAs are conserved targets of microRNAs. Genome Res 19:92-105

Gartel AL, Kandel ES (2006) RNA interference in cancer. Biomol Eng 23:17-34

Glud M, Manfe V, Biskup E, Holst L, Dirksen AM, Hastrup N, Nielsen FC, Drzewiecki KT, Gniadecki R (2011) MicroRNA miR-125b induces senescence in human melanoma cells. Melanoma Res 21:253-256

Gregory RI, Chendrimada TP, Cooch N, Shiekhattar R (2005) Human RISC couples microRNA biogenesis and posttranscriptional gene silencing. Cell 123:631-640

Gregory RI, Yan KP, Amuthan G, Chendrimada T, Doratotaj B, Cooch N, Shiekhattar R (2004) The Microprocessor complex mediates the genesis of microRNAs. Nature 432:235-240

Han J, Lee Y, Yeom KH, Kim YK, Jin H, Kim VN (2004) The Drosha-DGCR8 complex in primary microRNA processing. Genes Dev 18:3016-3027

Holst LM, Kaczkowski B, Gniadecki R (2010) Reproducible pattern of microRNA in normal human skin. Exp Dermatol 19:e201-205

Howell PM, Jr., Li X, Riker AI, Xi Y (2010) MicroRNA in Melanoma. Ochsner J 10:83-92

Kim BC, Seung NR, Park EJ, Kwon IH, Kim KH, Kim KJ, Park HR (2011) Immunohistochemical Study of the Expression of Astrocyte Elevated Gene-1 (AEG-1) in Malignant Melanoma, Spitz Nevus and Dysplastic Nevus. Korean J Dermatol 49::334-338

Kim VN (2004) MicroRNA precursors in motion: exportin-5 mediates their nuclear export. Trends Cell Biol 14:156-159

Landthaler M, Yalcin A, Tuschl T (2004) The human DiGeorge syndrome critical region gene 8 and Its D. melanogaster homolog are required for miRNA biogenesis. Curr Biol 14:2162-2167

Lee Y, Hur I, Park SY, Kim YK, Suh MR, Kim VN (2006) The role of PACT in the RNA silencing pathway. EMBO J 25:522-532

Lee Y, Jeon K, Lee JT, Kim S, Kim VN (2002) MicroRNA maturation: stepwise processing and subcellular localization. EMBO J 21:4663-4670

Lewis BP, Burge CB, Bartel DP (2005) Conserved seed pairing, often flanked by adenosines, indicates that thousands of human genes are microRNA targets. Cell 120:15-20

Li CL, Yang WZ, Chen YP, Yuan HS (2008) Structural and functional insights into human Tudor-SN, a key component linking RNA interference and editing. Nucleic Acids Res 36:3579-3589

Ma Z, Swede H, Cassarino D, Fleming E, Fire A, Dadras SS (2011) Up-regulated Dicer expression in patients with cutaneous melanoma. PLoS One 6:e20494

Mueller DW, Rehli M, Bosserhoff AK (2009) miRNA expression profiling in melanocytes and melanoma cell lines reveals miRNAs associated with formation and progression of malignant melanoma. J Invest Dermatol 129:1740-1751

Reinhart BJ, Slack FJ, Basson M, Pasquinelli AE, Bettinger JC, Rougvie AE, Horvitz HR, Ruvkun G (2000) The 21-nucleotide let-7 RNA regulates developmental timing in Caenorhabditis elegans. Nature 403:901-906

Riker AI, Enkemann SA, Fodstad O, Liu S, Ren S, Morris C, Xi Y, Howell P, Metge B, Samant RS, Shevde LA, Li W, Eschrich S, Daud A, Ju J, Matta J (2008) The gene expression profiles of primary and metastatic melanoma yields a transition point of tumor progression and metastasis. BMC Med Genomics 1:13

Sand M, Gambichler T, Sand D, Altmeyer P, Stuecker M, Bechara FG (2011a) Immunohistochemical expression patterns of the microRNA-processing enzyme Dicer in cutaneous malignant melanomas, benign melanocytic nevi and dysplastic melanocytic nevi. Eur J Dermatol 21:18-21

Sand M, Gambichler T, Sand D, Skrygan M, Altmeyer P, Bechara FG (2009) MicroRNAs and the skin: tiny players in the body's largest organ. J Dermatol Sci 53:169-175

Sand M, Gambichler T, Skrygan M, Sand D, Scola N, Altmeyer P, Bechara FG (2010) Expression levels of the microRNA processing enzymes Drosha and dicer in epithelial skin cancer. Cancer Invest 28:649-653

Sand M, Skrygan M, Georgas D, Arenz C, Gambichler T, Sand D, Altmeyer P, Bechara FG (2011b) Expression levels of the microRNA maturing microprocessor complex component DGCR8 and the RNA-induced silencing complex (RISC) components Argonaute-1, Argonaute-2, PACT, TARBP1, and TARBP2 in epithelial skin cancer. Mol Carcinog

Scatolini M, Grand MM, Grosso E, Venesio T, Pisacane A, Balsamo A, Sirovich R, Risio M, Chiorino G (2010) Altered molecular pathways in melanocytic lesions. Int J Cancer 126:1869-1881

Yoo BK, Santhekadur PK, Gredler R, Chen D, Emdad L, Bhutia S, Pannell L, Fisher PB, Sarkar D (2011) Increased RNA-induced silencing complex (RISC) activity contributes to hepatocellular carcinoma. Hepatology 53:1538-1548

Zhang JD, Biczok R, Ruschhaupt M (2011) http://www.bioconductor.org/packages/bioc/html/ddCt.html.

10 Paper 6: Immunohistochemical expression patterns of the microRNA-processing enzyme Dicer in cutaneous malignant melanomas, benign melanocytic nevi and dysplastic melanocytic nevi*

10.1 Introduction

MicroRNAs (miRNAs) are small endogenous molecules capable of post-transcriptional gene silencing [1]. Recently, miRNAs have been predicted to control approximately 30% of all genes in the human genome [2], and dysregulation of miRNAs has been demonstrated in a variety of malignant tumors [3]. Furthermore, miRNA metabolism in the skin and its appendages has been shown to be essential for normal skin morphogenesis. It is thus expected that disruption of proper miRNA expression can be observed in various malignant tumors, including malignant melanocytic skin lesions.

The microRNA-processing enzyme Dicer plays a central role in microRNA maturation and has been shown to be essential for skin morphogenesis [4]. Dicer is an RNase III enzyme that cleaves pre-miRNAs at a predetermined distance from the 3´ end, resulting in short fragments ranging from 21 to 27 nucleotides (nt) in length [5]. These mature miRNA strands can then be incorporated into the RNA-induced silencing complex (RISC), which is capable of modulating gene expression [6]. To date, 706 different mature miRNAs in humans have been described in the miRBase sequence database [7].

Recently the expression of microRNA-processing enzyme Dicer has shown to be downregulated in basal cell carcinoma and upregulated in squamous cell carcinoma of the skin [8]. However, there has been little investigation into the role of Dicer in melanocytic skin lesions. In order to further investigate the potential role of Dicer in benign or malignant melanocytic skin lesions, we conducted this pilot study examining immunohistochemical expression patterns of Dicer in cutaneous

---

* Co-authors: Thilo Gambichler M.D., Daniel Sand M.D., Peter Altmeyer M.D., Markus Stuecker M.D., Falk G. Bechara M.D.

malignant melanomas (CMM), benign melanocytic nevi (BMN), and dysplastic (DMN) melanocytic nevi.

10.2 Materials and Methods

This prospective pilot study was initiated at an academic university hospital and conducted within the framework of the Declaration of Helsinki. Informed consents were obtained from all study subjects. This study was approved by the Ethical Review Board of the Ruhr-University Bochum, Germany (registration number: 3265-08, ClinicalTrials.gov Identifier: NCT00862914).

10.2.1 Subjects

A total of 30 patients (17 females and 13 males with a median age of 52.4 ± 15.6 years) with benign melanocytic nevi (BMN, $n=10$), dysplastic melanocytic nevi (DMN, $n=10$), or cutaneous malignant melanomas (CMM, $n=10$) were enrolled in the study. Melanocytic skin lesions were excised with a scalpel under local anesthesia, and routine histologic examinations were performed. Non-lesional control specimens were harvested from adjacent healthy skin sites near tumor borders (intraindividual controls, $n=30$).

10.2.2 Immunohistochemistry

Skin specimens were fixed in 10% formalin, embedded in paraffin, and stained with haematoxylin and eosin. Four micrometer-thick sections were prepared and investigated by immunohistochemistry using commercially available mouse monoclonal anti-Dicer antibody (Clonegene cat #CG006, Hartford, CT). In order to ensure specificity of the antibody, endometrium specimen were used as a positive control according to the manufacturer guidelines. Briefly, paraffin sections were heated at 60°C for 12 hours and then deparaffinized in xylene and ethanol. Antigen retrieval was performed using 25 mmol/L of sodium citrate buffer (pH 6.0) at 90°C for 15 minutes, followed by treatment with 3% H_2O_2 to block endogenous peroxidase activity. The sections were then incubated with anti-Dicer antibody overnight in a moist chamber at 4°C. Sections were then rinsed in PBS, incubated with biotinylated goat anti-mouse immunoglobulin (Dako REAL™ Detection System, Alkaline Phosphatase/RED, Rabbit/Mouse, Code K5005) for 60 minutes at room temperature, and washed again in PBS. Reaction products were visualized with fast red chromogen using the Dako REAL™ Detection System. Color developed after 1.5-3 minutes, and the sections were washed in water, counterstained with haematoxylin, dehydrated, and mounted.

10.2.3 Quantitative Evaluation

Two observers (M.S. and F.G.B.) evaluated each section blind to patient clinical histories including the site of the lesion. Evaluation was performed with an ocular grid, counting only the positive reactions of melanocytes (expressed as the number per square area). Data were expressed as median per square millimeter.

Semiquantitative analysis was performed according to Klein et al. [9]. The expression index (EI) was determined by multiplying the area fraction of labeled cells (ALC) with the immunostaining intensity (ITI). ALC values were categorized into four scores: 0 = absence of labeled cells, 1 = 0-10% labeled cells, 2 = 11-50% labeled cells, 3 = > 50% labeled cells. The fractional area of labeled cells was determined using the following equation:

$$ALC = \frac{\text{total of counted labeled cells}}{500} \text{ x } 100 \rightarrow [\%]$$

We analyzed five dermal and five epidermal non-coincident microscopic fields at 400x magnification with a Leica DMLS light microscope and a 100-point grid. Labeled cells coinciding with grid points were counted. ITI was categorized with a score between 0 and 3 (0 = no staining, 1 = weak, 2 = moderate, 3 = strong intensity). Finally, EIs were calculated by multiplying the ALC and ITI (0 = no staining, 1-3 points = weak, 4 points = moderate, and 6-9 points = strong).

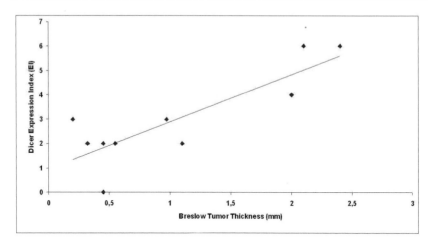

Fig. 10-1: X-Y-plot of the CMM Breslow tumor thickness (X-axis) and the CMM Dicer expression index (Y-axis) (r=0.84, p=0.022)

10.2.4 Statistical Analysis

Statistical analysis was performed using SPSS11.0 software. The null hypothesis was based on the assumption that there was no difference in Dicer ITI and EI scores between the three groups (BMN, DMN, CMM). Analysis of data distribution was assessed by the D`Agostino-Pearson test, and one-way ANOVA for three independent samples was performed for inter-arm comparisons. The Scheffe procedure for pair-wise comparisons was subsequently used to determine significant differences in ITI and EI scores reflecting Dicer expression. Mean differences and standard deviation (SD) of differences were calculated. Spearman correlation coefficient (r) was also analyzed. Statistical significance was set at 5% (two-sided).

10.3 Results

In the CMM group, the mean Breslow vertical tumor thickness was 1.05 mm (SD ± 0.82) with three Clark level II, three Clark level III and four Clark level IV. ITI scores for BMN, DMN and CMM were 0.9 (SD ± 0.57), 1.0 (SD ± 0.67), and 1.6 (SD ± 0.84), respectively. The mean corresponding EI scores were 1.3 (SD ± 1.16), 1.4 (SD ± 1.17), and 3.0 (SD ± 1.89), respectively. There was a significantly higher EI score for

Dicer in the CMM group compared to that in the BMN group ($p < 0.05$). However, EI differences between BMN and DMN as well as between CMM and DMN were not significant ($p > 0.05$). For CMM we observed a significant correlation of Breslow tumor thickness and EI (r=0.84, p=0.022) (Fig 10-1). Two BMN samples, two DMN samples, and one CMM sample showed very weak to no staining (EI score < 1).

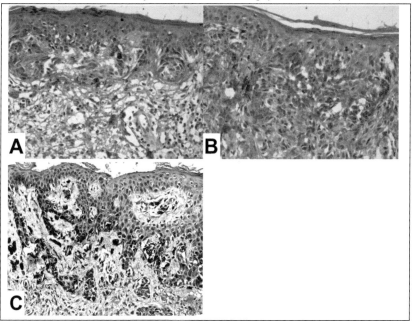

Fig. 10-2: Dicer expression in different melanocytic skin lesions. Immunoreactivity of Dicer is stronger in the dysplastic melanocytic nevi (A, ×400) and cutaneous malignant melanoma (B, ×400) (Breslow thickness, 2.1 mm; Clark level IV; T3aN0M0) compared with benign nevi (C, ×400).

Dicer-positive cells were primarily melanocytes and less keratinocytes and were also seen within the epidermal regions of BMN, DMN and CMM samples (Fig 10-2). Additionally, malignant melanocytes lying within tumor cell nests in dermal regions of CMM samples showed positive staining compared to the surrounding peritumoral stromal cells. The dermis showed only sparsely positive cells in addition to the malignant melanocytes. Positive staining was always cytoplasmic.

Healthy controls showed weak positive staining of epidermal keratinocytes and the basal lamina but was absent from the dermis.

Tab. 10-1: Number of lesion in each immunostaining intensity (ITI) category

ITI Scores	BMN	DMN	CMM
No staining (0)	2	2	1
Weak (1)	7	6	3
Moderate (2)	1	2	5
Strong (3)	0	0	1

Number of melanocytic skin lesion specimens listed for each immunostaining intensity (ITI) category. BMN, benign melanocytic nevi; DMN, dysplastic melanocytic nevi; CMM, cutaneous malignant melanomas.

Tab. 10-2: Number of lesion in each expression index (EI) category

EI Scores	BMN	DMN	CMM
No staining (0)	2	2	1
Weak (1-3)	7	7	6
Moderate (4)	1	1	1
Strong (6-9)	0	0	2

Number of melanocytic skin lesion specimens listed for each expression index (EI) category. BMN, benign melanocytic nevi; DMN, dysplastic melanocytic nevi; CMM, cutaneous malignant melanomas.

10.4 Discussion

Dicer is a key cytosolic regulator of miRNA maturation and a major component of the miRNA machinery. Alteration in Dicer and miRNA expression has been demonstrated in a variety of cancers [10]. Jakymiw et al. [11] demonstrated that Dicer protein expression is between 4- and 24-fold higher in head and neck squamous cell carcinoma (HNSCC) cell lines compared to normal gingival epithelial tissue. In the present pilot study, we performed immunohistochemical staining of benign and malignant melanocytic skin lesion samples embedded in paraffin to investigate Dicer expression as little is known about the role of miRNAs and its machinery in CMM, one of the most fatal malignancies [12]. Two recent studies from Mueller et al. and Kitago et al. have reported that a variety of specific miRNAs are dysregulated in cutaneous malignant melanomas which could account for changes in Dicer expression [13,14]. However, the few available studies investigating the potential role of miRNAs in melanoma pathogenesis were performed using melanoma cell lines and cultured melanocytes and did not pay attention to the miRNA machinery itself [15].

The intranuclear enzyme Drosha and the extracellular enzyme Dicer are essential parts of the miRNA machinery, which is responsible for cleaving pre-microRNAs into mature miRNAs [13,14]. Similar to previous studies that showed the central role for Dicer in skin morphogenesis, we found that Dicer was primarily expressed in the epidermis, which forms from the surface ectoderm of the embryo [16]. However, only a few sparse cells were Dicer-positive in the dermis, which is derived from the mesoderm or neural crest cells. It is possible that specific metabolic or genetic processes in epidermal cells require increased levels of miRNA maturation, which is reflected in the stronger epidermal staining. Although it is likely, one has to consider that altered Dicer expression is not explicit evidence for corresponding changes in the rate of miRNA maturation or increases in miRNA concentration within the cell. Other mechanisms than miRNA maturation through which Dicer could modify the cell behaviour have not been described. Therefore, further investigation is needed to clarify this issue.

Malignant melanocytes in CMM samples exhibited stronger Dicer expression compared to benign melanocytes and additionally to surrounding peritumoral stromal cells. As cancer cells have an altered metabolism, we were not surprised that Dicer expression appeared to be different in malignant melanocytes compared to benign melanocytes. Enhanced global transcription activity in melanoma cells could account for enhanced Dicer staining. However, we have to keep in mind that the differences in Dicer staining were not strong enough to differentiate between benign and malignant melanocytic proliferations. This shows that the role of dicer in melanoma may not be answered easily and that larger studies are necessary.

We found a significant positive correlation between Breslow tumor thickness and EI in the CMM group. We thus conclude that tumor-specific metabolism is probably associated with an increased demand for miRNA maturation.

Although this pilot study does not answer the question whether dicer expression per se have a tumor inducing effect we propose that we have a first indication for changes in Dicer expression which should be investigated with a larger sample size and an additional analysis of q-PCR data which was not undertaken because of financial and technical limitations.

Hence. the limitations of the present exploratory study include the small sample size and the absence of a second, independent method to verify our first results. We suggest that future studies examine a larger cohort as well as include another measure of Dicer expression, such as q-PCR of laser-microdissected epidermal, dermal and melanoma cells from paraffin or cryo-fixed tissue.

10.5 Conclusion

This pilot study presents preliminary evidence for possible differences in Dicer expression in malignant and benign melanocytes by immuno-histochemistry. Alterations in the miRNA machinery may play a role in the complex pathogenesis of melanomas and should be subject of further investigation.

10.6 References

1) Sand M, Gambichler T, Sand D, Skrygan M, Altmeyer P, Bechara FG. MicroRNAs and the skin: tiny players in the body's largest organ. J Dermatol Sci 2009;53:169-75.

2) Griffiths-Jones S, Saini HK, van Dongen S, Enright AJ. miRBase: tools for microRNA genomics. Nucleic Acids Res 2008;36:154-58.

3) Kanellopoulou C, Monticelli S. A role for microRNAs in the development of the immune system and in the pathogenesis of cancer. Semin Cancer Biol 2008;18:79-88.

4) Yi R, O'Carroll D, Pasolli HA, Zhang Z, Dietrich FS, Tarakhovsky A, Fuchs E. Morphogenesis in skin is governed by discrete sets of differentially expressed microRNAs. Nat Genet 2006;38:356–62.

5) Lee Y, Hur I, Park SY, Kim YK, Suh MR, Kim VN. The role of PACT in the RNA silencing pathway. EMBO J 2006;25:522-32.

6) Song JJ, Liu J, Tolia NH, Schneiderman J, Smith SK, Martienssen RA, Hannon GJ, Joshua-Tor L. The crystal structure of the Argonaute2 PAZ domain reveals an RNA binding motif in RNAi effector complexes. Nat Struct Biol 2003;10:1026-32.

7) miRNA database miRBase http://microrna.sanger.ac.uk/sequences/

8) Sand M, Gambichler T, Skrygan M, Sand D, Altmeyer P, Bechara FG. Expression levels of the microRNA processing enzymes Drosha and Dicer in epithelial skin cancer. Cancer Invest. 2010;28:649-53.

9) Klein M, Vignaud JM, Hennequin V, Toussaint B, Bresler L, Plénat F, Leclère J, Duprez A, Weryha G. Increased expression of the vascular endothelial growth factor is a pejorative prognosis marker in papillary thyroid carcinoma. J Clin Endocrinol Metab 2001;86:656-58.

10) Kanellopoulou C, Monticelli S. A role for microRNAs in the development of the immune system and in the pathogenesis of cancer. Semin Cancer Biol 2008;18:79-88.

11) Jakymiw A, Patel RS, Deming N, Bhattacharyya I, Shah P, Lamont RJ, Stewart CM, Cohen DM, Chan EK. Overexpression of dicer as a result of reduced let-7 MicroRNA levels contributes to increased cell proliferation of oral cancer cells. Genes Chromosomes Cancer 2010;49:549-59.

12) Geller AC, Swetter SM, Brooks K, Demierre MF, Yaroch AL. Screening, early detection, and trends for melanoma: current status (2000-2006) and future directions. J Am Acad Dermatol 2007;57:555-72.

13) Mueller DW, Rehli M, Bosserhoff AK. miRNA Expression Profiling in Melanocytes and Melanoma Cell Lines Reveals miRNAs Associated with Formation and Progression of Malignant Melanoma. J Invest Dermatol 2009;129:1740-51.

14) Kitago M, Martinez SR, Nakamura T, Sim MS, Hoon DS. Regulation of RUNX3 Tumor Suppressor Gene Expression in Cutaneous Melanoma. Clin Cancer Res 2009;15:2988-94.

15) Mueller DW, Bosserhoff AK. Integrin beta 3 expression is regulated by let-7a miRNA in malignant melanoma. Oncogene 2008;27:6698-706.

16) Andl T, Murchison EP, Liu F, Zhang Y, Yunta-Gonzalez M, Tobias JW, Andl CD, Seykora JT, Hannon GJ, Millar SE. The miRNA-processing enzyme dicer is essential for the morphogenesis and maintenance of hair follicles. Curr Biol 2006;16:1041-49.

11 Paper 7: Comparative microarray analysis of microRNA expression profiles in primary cutaneous malignant melanoma, cutaneous malignant melanoma metastases and benign melanocytic nevi[*]

11.1 Introduction

MicroRNAs (miRNA) are 17-25 nucleotide (nt) RNA molecules, which are capable of post-transcriptional gene regulation by binding to target mRNAs. Based on the degree of complementarity of the miRNA seed region between the nucleotides at positions 2 and 7 with the target mRNA, miRNA-mRNA binding can result in the translational repression or mRNA cleavage effectively silencing gene expression (Sand, et al., 2009). According to the current version of the miRNA database miRBase V.18, a total of 1527 different human miRNA sequences (out of approximately 3400 predicted miRNAs) have been described (miRBase, 2011, Sheng, et al., 2007). It has been estimated that 30 to 60 % of all human genes are potential targets of one or more miRNAs (Friedman, et al., 2009, Lewis, et al., 2005). With periodic updates of the miRNA database, miRBase, the list of human miRNAs identified is constantly growing. miRNA expression profiling studies based on updated versions of miRBase can facilitate the discovery of the involvement of newly added miRNAs that are included in updated versions of miRBase but not yet specifically linked to cutaneous malignant melanoma (CMM). Furthermore, miRNA expression profiling can independently validate the results of previous miRNA profiling studies. This study was undertaken to screen for differentially expressed miRNAs in primary cutaneous malignant melanoma (PCMM), cutaneous malignant melanoma metastases (CMMM) and benign melanocytic nevi (BMN) based on miRBase version 16 screening for 1205 human miRNAs in snap-frozen tumor specimens.

---

[*] Co-authors: Marina Skrygan Ph.D., Daniel Sand M.D., Dimitrios Georgas M.D., Thilo Gambichler M.D., Stephan Hahn, M.D., Peter Altmeyer M.D., Falk G. Bechara M.D.

11.2 Materials and Methods

This microRNA study was performed at the department of dermatological surgery at an academic university hospital (St. Josef Hospital, Ruhr University in Bochum, Germany).

This study was conducted within the framework of the declaration of Helsinki, and all tissues were taken with informed consent from the patients under a protocol approved by the Ethical Review Board of the Ruhr University in Bochum, Germany (registration number: 3265-08, ClinicalTrials.gov Identifier: NCT01482260).

11.2.1 Subjects

Twenty-one patients were enrolled in this study. Nine patients with PCMM were included, who were denoted PCMM1-PCMM9 and consisted of 2 females and 7 males with a median age of 76.3 years. Four patients with CMMM were included and were denoted CMMM1-CMMM4 and consisted of 2 females and 2 males with a median age of 74.3 years. Eight patients with congenital BMN were included and were denoted BMN1-BMN8 and consisted of 3 females and 5 males with a median age of 15.8 years. Patients with dysplastic nevi were excluded. Patient demographic details are shown in Tab. 11-1. All cutaneous specimens were harvested in the operating room, immediately submerged in RNAlater (Qiagen, Hilden, Germany) and kept at - 80 °C until RNA isolation.

11.2.2 RNA isolation

Total RNA including miRNAs was isolated using the miRNeasy Mini Kit (Qiagen, Hilden, Germany) according to the manufacturer's protocol. RNA concentration and purity were determined by using a NanoDrop ND-1000 spectrophotometer (Peqlab, Erlangen, Germany). RNA integrity (RIN) was determined by means of capillary electrophoresis using the 2100 Bioanalyzer and the RNA 6000 Nano LabChip kit (Agilent Technologies, Santa Clara, USA). The threshold for RNA quality suitable for microarray analysis was considered to be a RIN $\geq$ 7.0 indicating moderate to good RNA quality, as previously described by Thompson et al. (Thompson, et al., 2007).

11.2.3 Preparation of labeled miRNA, microarray hybridization and scanning

To assess the labeling and hybridization efficiencies, total RNA samples were spiked with synthesized oligonucleotides by using the MicroRNA Spike-In Kit (Agilent Technologies, Santa Clara, USA). A total of 100 ng of total RNA per sample was introduced into each labeling reaction. The spiked total RNA was treated with alkaline calf intestine phosphatase (CIP), and the resulting dephosphorylated RNA was labeled by using the miRNA Complete Labeling and Hyb Kit (Agilent Technologies, Santa Clara, USA) according to the manufacturer´s instructions using T4 RNA ligase to incorporate the dye Cyanine 3-Cytidine bisphosphate (pCp). The Cyanine 3-labeled miRNA samples were prepared for one-color based hybridization using the miRNA Complete Labeling and Hyb Kit (Agilent Technologies, Santa Clara, USA) according to the manufacturer´s instructions. Labeled miRNA samples were hybridized at 55°C for 20 hrs on human miRNA microarrays included in the Human miRNA Microarray Kit Release 16.0, 8x60K format (Agilent Technologies, Santa Clara, USA) screening for the expression of 1205 human miRNAs. After hybridization, the microarray slides were washed with increasing stringency using the Gene Expression Wash Buffers (Agilent Technologies, Santa Clara, USA), and the slides were dried with acetonitrile (Sigma-Aldrich, St. Louis, USA). Fluorescent signal intensities were detected using the Scan Control A.8.4.1 Software (Agilent Technologies, Santa Clara, USA) on the Agilent DNA Microarray Scanner and were extracted from the images using the Feature Extraction 10.7.3.1 Software (Agilent Technologies, Santa Clara, USA). All of the steps described regarding microarray processing were performed according to the manufacturer´s instructions.

Tab. 11-1: Details of the primary cutaneous malignant melanoma (PCMM), cutaneous malignant melanoma metastasis (CMMM) and benign melanocytic nevi (BMN) specimens included in this study. ALM=acral lentiginous melanoma, CL=Clark level, mm=millimeters, NMM=nodular malignant melanoma, RIN=RNA integrity number, SSM= superficial spreading melanoma, TT=tumor thickness.

Sample ID	Sex	Age	Locale	Histology	RNA conc. (ng/µl)	A260/280 ratio	RIN
PCMM_1	W	84	foot	unclassifiable melanoma, TT 3.2 mm, pT3	184.82	2.09	9.2
PCMM_2	M	73	epigastrium	NMM, TT 3.8 mm, CL IV, pT3b	444.22	1.92	9.2
PCMM_3	M	72	back	NMM, TT 2.1 mm, CL IV, pT3a	188.31	2.04	7.2
PCMM_4	M	76	lower leg	SSM, TT 3.2 mm, CL IV, pT3a	210.71	2.06	8.0
PCMM_5	M	84	back	SSM, TT 3.8 mm, CL IV, pT3a	331.66	2.07	7.5
PCMM_6	W	86	foot	ALM, TT 6.6 mm, CL IV, pT4b	139.56	2.07	7.4
PCMM_7	M	47	buttock	SSM, TT 2.1 mm, CL IV, pT3b	637.64	2.08	7.8
PCMM_8	M	86	lower leg	NMM, TT 1.4 mm, CL IV, pT2b	137.29	2.05	9.1
PCMM_9	M	79	popliteal fossa	NMM, TT 1.5 mm, CL IV, pT2a	96.64	2.07	8.9

Tab. 11-1: (Continued)

Sample ID	Sex	Age	Locale	Histology	RNA conc. (ng/µl)	A260/280 ratio	RIN
CMMM_1	W	70	thigh	CMMM	128.78	2.04	9.0
CMMM_2	M	76	thigh	CMMM	641.07	2.11	7.2
CMMM_3	W	82	medial ankle	CMMM	692.79	1.89	8.2
CMMM_4	M	69	iliac crest	CMMM	1518.82	2.03	6.9
BMN_1	W	13	flank	BMN	150.47	2.11	8.9
BMN_2	M	23	lower leg	BMN	69.38	2.02	8.5
BMN_3	M	9	upper arm	BMN	114.29	2.03	8.6
BMN_4	W	12	abdomen	BMN	117.55	2.06	8.6
BMN_5	M	25	shoulder	BMN	298.76	2.08	9.1
BMN_6	W	18	back of neck	BMN	62.33	2.06	7.7
BMN_7	M	16	shoulder	BMN	272.08	1.93	7.4
BMN_8	M	10	upper arm	BMN	412.29	1.90	7.0

11.2.4 Bioinformatic Data analyses

The data discussed in this study have been deposited in the National Center for Biotechnology Information (NCBI) Gene Expression Omnibus

(GEO) and are accessible through the GEO accession number GSE34460 (Internet address: http://www.ncbi.nlm.nih.gov/geo/query/ acc.cgi?acc=GSE34460) (Edgar, et al., 2002).

The software tools Feature Extraction 10.7.3.1, GeneSpring GX 11.5.1 (Agilent Technologies, Santa Clara, USA) and Spotfire Decision Site 9.1.2 (TIBCO Software Inc., Somerville, USA) were used for quality control, statistical data analysis, and miRNA annotation and visualization. Quantile normalization was applied to the data set to impose the same distribution of probe signal intensities for each array. The similarity between different samples based on global gene expression profiles was assessed by correlation analysis. Pearson's correlation coefficient (r) was calculated for all samples within the groups and for all pair-wise comparisons of the samples in this study. The Unweighted Pair-Group Method with Arithmetic Mean (UPGMA) clustering based on the Euclidean distance was applied to analyze the data (Sokal and Michener, 1958). The similarity measure used for the cluster analysis described in the present study was the "Euclidean distance" as previously described (Quackenbush, 2001). Hierarchical clustering was applied to the normalized data after filtering the data based on flags. After the normalized and log_2-transformed data were averaged across the replicates, the following pair-wise comparisons were analyzed:

1) The BMN group was used as the reference group, and miRNA expression of the combined cutaneous malignant melanoma group (PCMM + CMMM) was compared to this baseline.

2) The BMN group was used as the reference group, and miRNA expression of the PCMM group was compared to this baseline.

3) The CMMM group was used as the reference group, and miRNA expression of the PCMM group was compared to this baseline.

4) The nodular melanoma (NMM) subgroup (sample IDs PCMM2, PCMM3, PCMM8, PCMM9) was used as the reference group, and miRNA expression of the superficial spreading melanoma (SSM) subgroup (sample IDs PCMM4, PCMM5, PCMM7) was compared to this baseline.

11.2.5 Statistical analysis

Welch´s approximate t-test was applied to the comparisons made between the different groups. As the number of analyzed samples in this study was much lower than the number of hypotheses corresponding to the probes on the microarray chip, a substantial multiple testing error can occur. Therefore, the original p-values were adjusted to p-values for multiple testing by using a corrective algorithm devised by Benjamini and Hochberg (Benjamini and Hochberg, 1995).

The extent and direction of differential expression between the groups were determined by calculating the fold-change value. Normalized signal values were transformed from the $\log_2$ value to a linear scale, and their ratio was calculated. For the identification of differentially expressed miRNAs, the robustness of detection and the statistical significance were taken into account. Regarding statistical significance, a stringent filtering approach and a non-stringent filtering approach were used. For stringent filtering in the comparison of two groups, a miRNA was classified as induced if its corrected p-value was $\leq$ 0.05 with a fold-change value $\geq$ 2.0; a miRNA was considered repressed if its corrected p-value was $\leq$ 0.05 with a fold-change value $\geq$ - 2.0. For non-stringent filtering in a comparison of two groups, a miRNA was classified as induced if its non-adjusted p-value was $\leq$ 0.01 and 0.05 with a fold-change value $\geq$ 2.0; a miRNA was considered repressed if its non-adjusted p-value was $\leq$ 0.01 and 0.05 with a fold-change value $\geq$ - 2.0. For correlation analysis, the expression profiles of samples within and between the study groups were analyzed by determining Pearson´s correlation coefficient r.

11.2.6 Microarray data validation

The microarray data was validated by TaqMan quantitative real-time polymerase chain reaction (qRT-PCR). A group of 5 significantly up-regulated and 5 significantly down-regulated miRNA candidates and the reference gene snRNA U6 were chosen for qRT-PCR validation of the microarray data.

The TaqMan MicroRNA Reverse Transcription Kit (Applied Biosystems, Darmstadt, Germany) was used for the reverse transcription of the miRNA into single-stranded cDNA using assay-specific primers according to the manufacturer's instructions. For each miRNA that was verified, 10 ng of total RNA was reverse transcribed from each sample. qPCR analysis was performed in three technical replicates according to the manufacturer's instructions by using the TaqMan Universal Master Mix II no UNG (Applied Biosystems, Darmstadt, Germany) in a final reaction volume of 10 µl. The reaction mix was transferred into 384-well plates, and the plates were run on an AB7900HT qRT-PCR machine (Applied Biosystems, Darmstadt, Germany). The software SDS 2.4 (Applied Biosystems, Darmstadt, Germany) was used for instrument control, data acquisition and raw data analysis. The plates were run in relative quantification $(\Delta\Delta C_t)$ mode, and the following cycling temperature steps were used: 50°C for 2 min, 95°C for 10 min, then 40 cycles of 95°C for 15 s, then 60°C for 1 min. For data analysis, the cycle threshold C_t values were calculated using the software RQ Manager 1.2.1 (Applied Biosystems, Darmstadt, Germany). For qRT-PCR data analysis, the $\Delta\Delta C_t$ method, as previously described by Zhang et al., was used to calculate the relative expression levels of the target miRNAs (Zhang, et al., 2011). For correlative analysis of qRT-PCR and microarray results, the fold change values of the selected miRNAs were transformed to $\log_2$ values ($\log_2$(qPCR) and $\log_2$(microarray)). The Pearson´s correlation coefficient, as well as a paired two-tailed t-test was calculated for each comparison made with a significance cutoff value set at $p < 0.05$.

11.2.7 Mining data analysis

The human miRNA-associated disease database HMDD (http://cmbi. bjmu.edu.cn/hmdd), the miRNA database for miRNA functional annotations miRDB (http://mirdb.org/miRDB), the Mir2Disease database (http://www.mir2disease.org/) (Jiang, et al., 2009), the Melanoma Molecular Map project (http://www.mmmp.org/MMMP/) and PubMed (http://www.ncbi.nlm.nih.gov/pubmed/) were used to identify and compare previously described associations between differentially expressed miRNAs in cutaneous melanoma with associations observed in the present study.

11.3 Results

11.3.1 Quality control

Quality control (QC) reports were generated by using the Feature Extraction software 10.7.3.1 (Agilent Technologies, Santa Clara, USA) for each individual array, and it was verified that all quality criteria for microarray analysis were fulfilled by all samples included in this study. Additional visual control of probes spotted on the corners of the chip were compared to the QC reports and confirmed the accuracy of automatic corner finding and grid placing for all arrays in this study.

11.3.2 Correlation analysis

The correlation analysis within the groups revealed moderate correlation coefficients. Within the PCMM group, the r-values ranged from 0.832 to 0.963 with an average r-value of 0.918. Within the PCMM subgroup NMM, the r-values ranged from 0.89 to 0.941 with an average r-value of 0.917. Within the PCMM subgroup SSM, the r-values ranged from 0.935 to 0.955 with an average r-value of 0.947. Within the CMMM group, the r-values ranged from 0.853 to 0.938 with an average r-value of 0.905. Within the BMN group, the r-values ranged from 0.926 to 0.988 with an average r-value of 0.96.

When analyzing differences among the groups, the correlation coefficients indicated a moderate correlation. The correlation coefficients between the combined melanoma group (PCMM + CMMM) and the BMN group ranged from 0.823 to 0.96 with an average r-value of 0.917. Correlation coefficients between the PCMM subgroup NMM and the BMN group ranged from 0.864 to 0.959 with an average r-value of 0.92. The correlation coefficients between the PCMM subgroup SSM and the BMN group ranged from 0.905 to 0.958 with an average r-value of 0.938. The correlation coefficients between the PCMM group and the CMMM group ranged from 0.847 to 0.961 with an average r-value of 0.911. The correlation coefficients between the PCMM subgroup NMM and the CMMM group ranged from 0.864 to 0.953 with an average r-value of 0.913. The correlation coefficients between the PCMM subgroup SSM and the CMMM group ranged from 0.878 to 0.961 with an average r-value of 0.928. The correlation coefficients between the PCMM subgroup NMM and the PCMM subgroup SSM ranged from 0.907 to 0.963 with an average r-value of 0.937. The correlation coefficients between the BMN group and the CMMM group ranged from 0.823 to 0.948 with an average r-value of 0.906. For details on the correlation analysis, see Fig. 11-1 and Tab. 11-2.

11.3.3 Cluster analysis

Hierarchical clustering of normalized data showed a very high degree of similarity between the samples across all three groups (Fig. 11-2). An analysis of the heat map did not reveal clusters between the different groups, as the samples in this study showed very heterogeneous miRNA expression profiles. CMMM3 proved to be the most significantly different sample regarding miRNA expression when compared to the twenty other samples in this study (Fig. 11-2).

11.3.4 Differential miRNA expression

When comparing the miRNA expression profiles of the PCMM and CMMM groups with the expression profiles of the BMN group using a stringent filtering approach, 22 upregulated and 28 downregulated miRNAs were identified. With respect to fold-change, the ten most upregulated miRNAs were hsa-miR-18a, hsa-miR-18b, hsa-miR-21*, hsa-miR-142-3p, hsa-miR-155, hsa-miR-223, hsa-miR-301a, hsa-miR-484, hsa-miR-663 and hsa-miR-1274a. The ten most downregulated miRNAs were hsa-miR-24-1*, hsa-miR-149, hsa-miR-183, hsa-miR-200a, hsa-miR-200b, hsa-miR-204, hsa-miR-224*, hsa-miR-429, hsa-miR-455-5p and hsa-miR-664. Comparing the miRNA expression profile of the PCMM samples to the expression profile of the BMN samples revealed hsa-miR-21*, hsa-miR-155, hsa-miR-142-3p, hsa-miR-21, hsa-miR-3663-3p, hsa-miR-4281, hsa-miR-720 and hsa-miR-4286 to be the most upregulated and hsa-let-7a, hsa-miR-23b, hsa-miR-24-1*, hsa-miR-125b, hsa-miR-149, hsa-miR-183, hsa-miR-200a, hsa-miR-204, hsa-miR-429, hsa-miR-455-5p, hsa-miR-574-3p and hsa-miR-664 to be the most downregulated miRNAs.

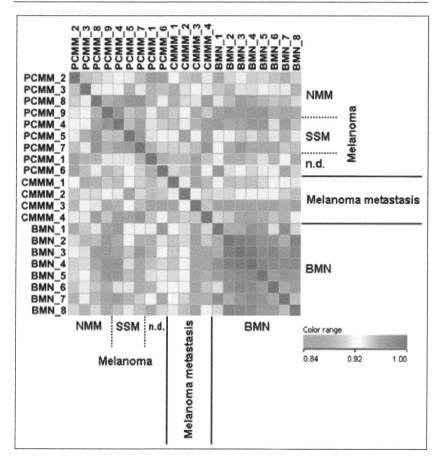

Fig. 11-1:   Heat map plot for the correlation coefficients r. The color scale on the right side reflects the correlation of samples and ranges from green, which indicates a moderate correlation, to red, which indicates a high correlation.
PCMM=primary cutaneous malignant melanoma,
CMMM=cutaneous malignant melanoma metastases,
BMN=benign melanocytic nevi.

Tab. 11-2: Correlation matrix of all PCMM, CMMM and BMN samples (averaged values are shown in blue)

Group		Group 1 (PCMM)									
Sub-Group		NMM				SSM			n.d.		
Group	Sub-Group	Sample Name	PCMM_2	PCMM_3	PCMM_8	PCMM_9	PCMM_4	PCMM_5	PCMM_7	PCMM_1	PCMM_6
Group 1 (PCMM)	NMM	PCMM_2	1.000								
		PCMM_3	0.890	1.000							
		PCMM_8	0.932	0.922	1.000						
		PCMM_9	0.904	0.911	0.941	1.000 *(0.917)*					
	SSM	PCMM_4	0.915	0.913	0.948	0.960	1.000				
		PCMM_5	0.907	0.942	0.958	0.935	0.935	1.000			
		PCMM_7	0.936	0.923	0.963	0.941	0.949	0.955	1.000 *(0.947)*		
	n.d.	PCMM_1	0.832	0.880	0.881	0.923	0.906	0.904	0.881	1.000	
		PCMM_6	0.841	0.888	0.909	0.939	0.933	0.911	0.898	0.942	1.000 *(0.918)*

Averaged (blue) values: NMM = 0.917; NMM_SSM = 0.937; SSM = 0.947; n.d. = 0.918

Tab. 11-2: (Continued)

Group	Sub-Group	Sample Name	Group 2 (CMMM) — n.d.				Group 3 (BMN) — n.d.							
			CMMM_1	CMMM_2	CMMM_3	CMMM_4	BMN_1	BMN_2	BMN_3	BMN_4	BMN_5	BMN_6	BMN_7	BMN_8
Group 1 (PCMM)	NMM	PCMM_2				PCMM_ CMMM 0.911								PCMM_BMN 0.923
		PCMM_3		NMM_ CMMM 0.913						NMM_BMN 0.920				
		PCMM_8												
		PCMM_9												
	SSM	PCMM_4		SSM_ CMMM 0.928						SSM_BMN 0.938				
		PCMM_5												
		PCMM_7												
	n.d.	PCMM_1								0.917				
		PCMM_6												

Tab. 11-2: (Continued)

Group	Sub-Group	Sample Name	NMM				SSM			n.d.	
			PCMM_2	PCMM_3	PCMM_8	PCMM_9	PCMM_4	PCMM_5	PCMM_7	PCMM_1	PCMM_6
Group 2 (CMMM)	n.d.	CMMM_1	0.912	0.869	0.941	0.933	0.937	0.915	0.931	0.886	0.899
		CMMM_2	0.891	0.926	0.928	0.918	0.922	0.950	0.929	0.887	0.891
		CMMM_3	0.880	0.911	0.905	0.864	0.878	0.919	0.887	0.847	0.849
		CMMM_4	0.923	0.923	0.953	0.934	0.953	0.949	0.961	0.891	0.911
Group 3 (BMN)	n.d.	BMN_1	0.864	0.892	0.924	0.949	0.956	0.915	0.920	0.922	0.960
		BMN_2	0.899	0.880	0.936	0.956	0.945	0.913	0.944	0.875	0.902
		BMN_3	0.909	0.903	0.954	0.955	0.949	0.934	0.958	0.872	0.911
		BMN_4	0.894	0.901	0.947	0.959	0.958	0.927	0.947	0.888	0.929
		BMN_5	0.898	0.911	0.939	0.959	0.958	0.937	0.947	0.903	0.923
		BMN_6	0.890	0.907	0.934	0.943	0.927	0.924	0.945	0.879	0.908
		BMN_7	0.876	0.923	0.938	0.948	0.953	0.941	0.933	0.911	0.948
		BMN_8	0.896	0.875	0.930	0.946	0.937	0.905	0.937	0.863	0.895

Tab. 11-2: (Continued)

Group	Sub-Group	Sample Name	CMMM_1	CMMM_2	CMMM_3	CMMM_4	BMN_1	BMN_2	BMN_3	BMN_4	BMN_5	BMN_6	BMN_7	BMN_8
Group 2 (CMMM)	n.d.	CMMM_1	1.000											
		CMMM_2	0.908	1.000										
		CMMM_3	0.853	0.910	1.000									
		CMMM_4	0.938	0.931	0.892	1.000								
Group 3 (BMN)	n.d.	BMN_1	0.915	0.902	0.852	0.929	1.000							
		BMN_2	0.937	0.898	0.831	0.932	0.943	1.000						
		BMN_3	0.935	0.921	0.854	0.947	0.943	0.981	1.000					
		BMN_4	0.935	0.919	0.851	0.948	0.962	0.980	0.988	1.000				
		BMN_5	0.929	0.915	0.854	0.943	0.954	0.963	0.968	0.972	1.000			
		BMN_6	0.917	0.913	0.846	0.935	0.926	0.960	0.973	0.966	0.953	1.000		
		BMN_7	0.919	0.931	0.873	0.942	0.968	0.942	0.958	0.967	0.959	0.945	1.000	
		BMN_8	0.925	0.885	0.823	0.922	0.931	0.983	0.977	0.972	0.957	0.955	0.938	1.000

CMMM_4: 0.905

PCMM+CMMM_BMN

MMM_BMN: 0.906 / 0.960

Comparing PCMM and CMMM using a non-stringent filtering approach, we found that hsa-miR-1, hsa-miR-17*, hsa-miR-31, hsa-miR-31*, hsa-miR-145*, hsa-miR-486-5p, hsa-miR-4291, and hsa-miR-4317 were upregulated and that hsa-miR-15b, hsa-miR-34c-5p, hsa-miR-148a, hsa-miR-424 and hsa-miR-542-5p were downregulated. When comparing the PCMM subgroup SSM and the NMM group, we found that hsa-miR-664* and hsa-miR-766 were upregulated and no miRNAs were significantly downregulated. The detailed report of the differentially expressed miRNAs in the different groups is shown in Tab. 11-3 and 11-4.

11.3.5 RT-PCR Validation

The microarray data was validated by TaqMan real-time reverse transcription polymerase chain reaction (RT-PCR). We choose a group of 5 upregulated (hsa-miR-21, hsa-miR-142-3p, hsa-miR-155, hsa-miR-223, and hsa-miR-301a) and 5 down-regulated (hsa-miR-141, hsa-miR-149, hsa-miR-200b, hsa-miR-204, and hsa-miR-455-3p) miRNAs and the reference gene snRNA U6 for TaqMan RT-PCR validation. Fig. 11-3 summarizes the differential expression between the BMN group and the PCMM+CMMM group. Pearson´s correlation coefficient r and the p-value based on the paired two-tailed t-test were calculated using the $\log_2$ fold-change values from the qPCR and microarray results of the analyzed miRNAs identified above. Pearson´s correlation coefficient r was calculated to be 0.956 (BMN vs. PCMM+CMMM) with a p-value of 0.135 (BMN vs. PCMM+CMMM) showing a very high correlation between the qPCR and microarray results for the comparison of BMN vs. PCMM+CMMM (Fig. 11-4).

11.3.6 Data mining results

The miRNAs that have not previously been associated with CMM and that were differentially expressed included fourteen upregulated and five downregulated miRNA candidates. The upregulated miRNA candidates included hsa-miR-22, hsa-miR-130b, hsa-miR-146b-5p, hsa-miR-223, hsa-miR-301a, hsa-miR-484, hsa-miR-663, hsa-miR-720, hsa-miR-1260, hsa-miR-1274a, hsa-miR-1274b, hsa-miR-3663-3p, hsa-miR-4281 and hsa-miR-4286. The down-regulated miRNAs included hsa-miR-24-1*, hsa-miR-26a, hsa-miR-4291, hsa-miR-4317 and hsa-miR-4324. Several miRNAs were identified as significantly differentially expressed, and these are discussed in the following section.

11.4 Discussion

miRNAs participate in multiple fundamental and diverse cellular processes, such as gene regulation, gene expression, cell differentiation, cell proliferation and apoptosis. Their role in primary cutaneous malignant melanoma (PCMM) and cutaneous malignant melanoma metastasis (CMMM) development and progression has recently attracted a lot of attention (Ambros, 2004, Bartel, 2004, Howell, et al., 2010, Karube, et al., 2005, Lee, et al., 2005, Takamizawa, et al., 2004). A variety of studies have been undertaken to investigate possible perturbations in the miRNA machinery itself and to describe the differences in the miRNA expression profiles of melanoma cell lines and fresh melanoma tissue compared to normal melanocytes (Bonazzi, et al., 2011, Sand, et al., 2011, Sand, et al., 2012).

Clinically, PCMM is by far the most deadly and aggressive form of skin cancer, as it is often associated with a poor prognosis and a lack of effective, standardized therapies in the case of advanced disease (Mueller and Bosserhoff, 2009). As a consequence, basic scientific research investigating the possible role of differentially expressed miRNAs in PCMM and CMMM formation or progression is needed to identify novel biomarkers and novel forms of miRNA-based gene therapy options.

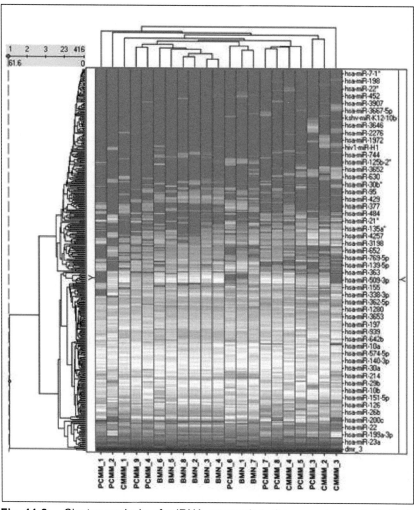

Fig. 11-2: Cluster analysis of miRNA expression shows a strong similarity to the expression data in the heat map with 416 filtered miRNAs. The color scale reflects the signal intensity converted to log2 and ranges from red, which indicates a low intensity, to white, which indicates a moderate intensity, to blue, which indicates a strong intensity. The dendrogram on the left reflects the hierarchical similarity. The cluster slider above the dendrogram consists of two scales. The upper scale shows the number of clusters at different positions in the dendrogram. The lower scale shows the calculated similarity score for the different positions in the dendrogram.

Tab. 11-3: Total numbers of differentially expressed miRNAs for each group comparison. The first column displays the adjusted p value (adj.-p), the second and third columns display the non-adjusted p-values (p). Primary cutaneous malignant melanoma (PCMM), cutaneous malignant melanoma metastases (CMMM), benign melanocytic nevi (BMN), fold change (FC)

Comparison	adj.-p ≤ 0.05 $|FC| \geq 2.0$		p ≤ 0.01 $|FC| \geq 2.0$		p ≤ 0.05 $|FC| \geq 2.0$	
	Up	Down	Up	Down	Up	Down
[PCMM+CMMM] vs. BMN	21	28	21	29	36	52
PCMM vs. BMN	8	12	16	22	29	39
PCMM vs. CMMM	0	1	3	1	9	5
SSM vs. NMM	0	0	1	0	2	0

Previously, a variety of specific miRNAs in different stages of PCMM development and progression have been described as dysregulated. Among the miRNAs specifically described in the literature as significantly increased and associated with PCMM development include hsa-miR-106, hsa-miR-126, hsa-miR-133a, hsa-miR-141, hsa-miR-145, hsa-miR-15b, hsa-miR-200c, hsa-miR-210 and hsa-miR-27b (Molnar, et al., 2008, Mueller, et al., 2009, Satzger, et al., 2010, Zhang, et al., 2009). On the other hand, the miRNAs hsa-let-7a, hsa-let-7b, hsa-miR-155, hsa-miR324-5p and hsa-miR-34a have been repeatedly described as significantly downregulated in the PCMM development process (Levati, et al., 2009, Molnar, Tamasi, Bakos, Wiener and Falus, 2008, Mueller, Rehli and Bosserhoff, 2009, Muller and Bosserhoff, 2008, Satzger, Mattern, Kuettler, Weinspach, Voelker, Kapp and Gutzmer, 2010, Schultz, et al., 2008). For a detailed list of the representative miRNAs that are currently known to be involved in the different progression stages of PCMM, refer to the reviews of Bonazzi et al. and Howell et al. (Bonazzi, Stark and Hayward, 2011, Howell, Li, Riker and Xi, 2010).

Our miRNA profiling study is the first to use fresh frozen clinical PCMM and CMMM specimens, as well as an Agilent platform with miRBase version 16. Therefore, we expected to find previously described differentially expressed miRNA genes as well as novel miRNA candidates not yet associated with CMM. The novel miRNA candidates include hsa-miR-301a, an activator of the transcriptional factor nuclear factor κB (NF-κB). In human pancreas cancer cells, hsa-miR-301a overexpression leads to increased NF-κB activation by the down-regulation of the NF-κB repressing factor Nκrf (Lu, et al., 2011). It has also been shown that NF-κB is up-regulated in human CMM leading to the dysregulation of gene transcription (Ueda and Richmond, 2006). Whether hsa-miR-301a-induced activation of NF-κB is also relevant for CMM development will be an interesting future investigation. Hsa-miR-130b is another newly identified candidate, which has been shown to target tumor protein p53-inducible nuclear protein 1 (*TP53INP1*) (Yeung, et al., 2008). The decreased expression of *TP53INP1* has been previously reported in CMM, which makes the investigation of the role of hsa-miR-130b in CMM an interesting topic (Bonazzi, et al., 2009, Sigalotti, et al., 2010). Hsa-miR-146b-5p suppresses epidermal growth factor receptor (*EGFR*) expression and binds to *SMAD4*, an important member of the transforming growth factor β (*TGF-β*) signaling pathway (Geraldo, et al., 2011, Katakowski, et al., 2010). EGFR has been shown to be increased in CMM cell lines and to be involved in the progression and metastasis of a subset of CMM (Boone, et al., 2011, de Wit, et al., 1992). *TGF-β* has received a considerable amount of attention in the study of the molecular pathogenesis of CMM, as it has multiple tumor-promoting effects (Busse and Keilholz, 2011). Whether the modulation of *EGFR* or the *TGF-β* pathway by miR-146b-5p plays a role in CMM tumorigenesis warrants further investigation. Hsa-miR-26a was downregulated in the CMM group in our study, and this miRNA has previously been shown to target the enhancer of zeste homolog 2

(*EZH2*), which is a cell cycle regulator and epigenetic transcriptional repressor (Sander, et al., 2008). *EZH2* has been proposed to play a role in CMM pathogenesis and progression, as it leads to enhanced tumorigenicity through the repression of p21 (Fan, et al., 2011, McHugh, et al., 2007). Therefore, it would be interesting to examine whether the increased EZH2 expression in CMM could be due to hsa-mir-26a down-regulation.

The differentially expressed miRNAs in this study that have been previously reported to associate with CMM include hsa-mir-155, which has been reported to be significantly elevated in PCMM samples by several other authors (Lesinski, et al., 2008, Philippidou, et al., 2010, Segura, et al., 2010). Hsa-mir-155 is another miRNA that has been shown to be upregulated in a variety of other cancers, such as thyroid, breast, colon, cervical and lung cancers (Faraoni, et al., 2009). The down-regulation of hsa-mir-155 has also been reported; however, this particular study was performed on melanoma cell lines and not on fresh clinical melanoma specimens. The discrepancy in reports appears to be a cell culture-related phenomenon (Levati, Alvino, Pagani, Arcelli, Caporaso, Bondanza, Di Leva, Ferracin, Volinia, Bonmassar, Croce and D'Atri, 2009, Mueller and Bosserhoff, 2011).

Hsa-mir-18a associates with the hsa-mir-17-92 cluster, also known as Oncomir-1, which consists of 6 miRNA members (hsa-mir-17, hsa-mir-18a, hsa-mir-19a, hsa-mir-19b-1, hsa-mir-20a and hsa-mir-92). Hsa-mir-18b associates with the miRNA cluster, miR-106-363, which also consists of 6 members (hsa-mir-106a, hsa-mir-18b, hsa-mir-20b, hsa-mir-19b-2, hsa-mir-92a-2 and hsa-mir-363). Both hsa-mir-18a and hsa-mir-18b have previously been shown to be associated with CMM (Howell, Li, Riker and Xi, 2010, Leidinger, et al., 2010).

Tab. 11-4: Significantly dysregulated miRNAs arranged by their fold change (FC). PCMM=primary cutaneous malignant melanoma, CMMM= cutaneous malignant melanoma metastases, BMN= benign melanocytic nevi, SSM= superficial spreading melanoma, NMM=nodular melanoma, **bold**= not previously associated with cutaneous melanoma, *italics*= previously associated with cutaneous melanoma

Comparison	miRNA	Fold-change	Corrected p-value	Citation
[PCMM+CMMM] **vs.** **BMN**	*hsa-miR-21**	79.48583	3.40E-05	(Grignol, et al., 2011, Jiang, et al., 2009)
	hsa-miR-301a	14.670435	0.01550083	
	hsa-miR-155	11.204804	0.02728053	(Faraoni, et al., 2009, Levati, et al., 2009)
	hsa-miR-663	10.240385	0.041589	
	hsa-miR-18a	8.2596445	0.0384784	(Howell, et al., 2010, Leidinger, et al., 2010)
	hsa-miR-18b	7.2364845	0.02728053	(Howell, Li, Riker and Xi, 2010)
	hsa-miR-484	6.1434307	0.02730224	
	hsa-miR-142-3p	4.8376527	0.00494103	(Chan, et al., 2011, Leidinger, Keller, Borries, Reichrath, Rass, Jager, Lenhof and Meese, 2010)
	hsa-miR-1274a	4.4074693	0.00612403	
	hsa-miR-223	4.377534	0.0291837	
	hsa-miR-21	4.1862392	0.00612403	(Xu, et al., 2012)

adjusted p-value ≤ 0.05, fold change ≥ 2.0 — Up

Tab. 11-4: (Continued)

Comparison	adjusted p-value ≤ 0.05, fold change ≥ 2.0 Up			
	miRNA	Fold-change	Corrected p-value	Citation
[PCMM+CMMM] vs. BMN	hsa-miR-1274b	2.7395546	0.00612403	(Leidinger, Keller, Borries, Reichrath, Rass, Jager, Lenhof and Meese, 2010)
	hsa-miR-4281	2.5769475	0.01024456	
	hsa-miR-130b	2.5270877	0.01060002	
	hsa-miR-3663-3p	2.4002712	0.00592998	
	hsa-miR-720	2.3566184	0.00023395	
	hsa-miR-4286	2.2943316	0.00408535	
	hsa-miR-146b-5p	2.2454796	0.03745918	
	hsa-miR-1260	2.14991	0.00592998	
	hsa-miR-1280	2.058045	0.02419796	
	hsa-miR-22	2.0233924	0.0384784	

Tab. 11-4: (Continued)

| Comparison | adjusted p-value ≤ 0.05, fold change ≥ 2.0 | | | |
| | Down | | | |
	miRNA	Fold-change	Corrected p-value	Citation
[PCMM+CMMM] vs. BMN	hsa-miR-429	-106.252625	1.04E-08	(Xu, Brenn, Brown, Doherty and Melton, 2012, Zhang, et al., 2006)
	hsa-miR-200a	-50.146927	0.00139825	(Gaur, et al., 2007, Xu, Brenn, Brown, Doherty and Melton, 2012, Zhang, Huang, Yang, Greshock, Megraw, Giannakakis, Liang, Naylor, Barchetti, Ward, Yao, Medina, O'Brien-Jenkins, Katsaros, Hatzigeorgiou, Gimotty, Weber and Coukos, 2006)
	hsa-miR-455-5p	-39.76875	0.01328589	(Jukic, et al., 2010, Xu, Brenn, Brown, Doherty and Melton, 2012)
	hsa-miR-204	-35.481976	0.00612403	(Yang and Wei, 2011)
	hsa-miR-149	-24.936562	0.00494103	(Xu, Brenn, Brown, Doherty and Melton, 2012)

Tab. 11-4: (Continued)

Comparison	adjusted p-value ≤ 0.05, fold change ≥ 2.0 Down			
	miRNA	Fold-change	Corrected p-value	Citation
[PCMM+CMMM] vs. BMN	hsa-miR-183	-23.152014	0.0003439	(Xu, Brenn, Brown, Doherty and Melton, 2012, Zhang, Huang, Yang, Greshock, Megraw, Giannakakis, Liang, Naylor, Barchetti, Ward, Yao, Medina, O'Brien-Jenkins, Katsaros, Hatzigeorgiou, Gimotty, Weber and Coukos, 2006)
	hsa-miR-664	-17.891062	0.00231677	(Leidinger, Keller, Borries, Reichrath, Rass, Jager, Lenhof and Meese, 2010)
	hsa-miR-24-1*	-13.43965	0.00698503	
	hsa-miR-200b	-12.465944	0.02536456	(Gaur, Jewell, Liang, Ridzon, Moore, Chen, Ambros and Israel, 2007, Xu, Brenn, Brown, Doherty and Melton, 2012, Zhang, Huang, Yang, Greshock, Megraw, Giannakakis, Liang, Naylor, Barchetti, Ward, Yao, Medina, O'Brien-Jenkins, Katsaros, Hatzigeorgiou, Gimotty, Weber and Coukos, 2006)

Tab. 11-4: (Continued)

Comparison		adjusted p-value ≤ 0.05, fold change ≥ 2.0		
		Down		
[PCMM+CMMM] vs. BMN	miRNA	Fold-change	Corrected p-value	Citation
	hsa-miR-224*	-12.329998	0.02728053	(Xu, Brenn, Brown, Doherty and Melton, 2012, Zhang, Huang, Yang, Greshock, Megraw, Giannakakis, Liang, Naylor, Barchetti, Ward, Yao, Medina, O'Brien-Jenkins, Katsaros, Hatzigeorgiou, Gimotty, Weber and Coukos, 2006)
	hsa-miR-141	-11.41825	0.04526546	
	hsa-miR-200c	-11.207425	0.04350069	(Gaur, Jewell, Liang, Ridzon, Moore, Chen, Ambros and Israel, 2007, Xu, Brenn, Brown, Doherty and Melton, 2012, Zhang, Huang, Yang, Greshock, Megraw, Giannakakis, Liang, Naylor, Barchetti, Ward, Yao, Medina, O'Brien-Jenkins, Katsaros, Hatzigeorgiou, Gimotty, Weber and Coukos, 2006)
	hsa-miR-4291	-9.461466	0.02318372	

Tab. 11-4: (Continued)

Comparison		adjusted p-value ≤ 0.05, fold change ≥ 2.0		
		Down		
	miRNA	Fold-change	Corrected p-value	Citation
[PCMM+CMMM] vs. BMN	hsa-miR-224	-9.347525	0.02419796	(Xu, Brenn, Brown, Doherty and Melton, 2012)
	hsa-miR-4324	-8.964951	0.01328191	
	hsa-miR-23b*	-8.806605	0.00777689	
	hsa-miR-4317	-8.454064	0.00777689	
	hsa-miR-192	-6.6436357	0.04762697	(Caramuta, et al., 2010)
	hsa-miR-29c*	-5.7982626	0.04055328	(Jukic, Rao, Kelly, Skaf, Drogowski, Kirkwood and Panelli, 2010)
	hsa-miR-455-3p	-3.6730921	0.00494103	(Segura, et al., 2010, Xu, Brenn, Brown, Doherty and Melton, 2012)
	hsa-miR-186	-3.5160537	0.02786352	(Leidinger, Keller, Borries, Reichrath, Rass, Jager, Lenhof and Meese, 2010, Zhang, Huang, Yang, Greshock, Megraw, Giannakakis, Liang, Naylor, Barchetti, Ward, Yao, Medina, O'Brien-Jenkins, Katsaros, Hatzigeorgiou, Gimotty, Weber and Coukos, 2006)

Tab. 11-4: (Continued)

Comparison	miRNA	Fold-change	Corrected p-value	Citation
[PCMM+CMMM] vs. BMN		adjusted p-value ≤ 0.05, fold change ≥ 2.0 Down		
	hsa-miR-574-3p	-3.3989756	0.00231677	(Jukic, Rao, Kelly, Skaf, Drogowski, Kirkwood and Panelli, 2010)
	hsa-miR-23b	-3.1663396	0.00231677	(Philippidou, et al., 2010, Satzger, et al., 2010)
	hsa-miR-100	-2.8878741	0.00683224	(Zhang, Huang, Yang, Greshock, Megraw, Giannakakis, Liang, Naylor, Barchetti, Ward, Yao, Medina, O'Brien-Jenkins, Katsaros, Hatzigeorgiou, Gimotty, Weber and Coukos, 2006)
	hsa-miR-27b	-2.3595865	0.00494103	(Philippidou, Schmitt, Moser, Margue, Nazarov, Muller, Vallar, Nashan, Behrmann and Kreis, 2010)
	hsa-miR-125b	-2.3502712	0.03217045	(Glud, et al., 2010)
	hsa-let-7a	-2.061917	0.00139175	(Muller and Bosserhoff, 2008)
	hsa-miR-26a	-2.0184028	0.00231677	

Tab. 11-4:   (Continued)

| Comparison | adjusted p-value ≤ 0.05, fold change ≥ 2.0 | | | |
| | mirNA | Up | | |
		Fold-change	Corrected p-value	Citation
PCMM vs. BMN	hsa-miR-21*	69.10735	0.01186657	(Jiang, Wang, Hao, Juan, Teng, Zhang, Li, Wang and Liu, 2009, Yang, et al., 2011)
	hsa-miR-155	13.59634	0.04377073	(Faraoni, Antonetti, Cardone and Bonmassar, 2009, Levati, Alvino, Pagani, Arcelli, Caporaso, Bondanza, Di Leva, Ferracin, Volinia, Bonmassar, Croce and D'Atri, 2009)
	hsa-miR-142-3p	4.156645	0.02128333	(Chan, Patel, Nallur, Ratner, Bacchiocchi, Hoyt, Szpakowski, Godshalk, Ariyan, Sznol, Halaban, Krauthammer, Tuck, Slack and Weidhaas, 2011, Leidinger, Keller, Borries, Reichrath, Rass, Jager, Lenhof and Meese, 2010)

Tab. 11-4: (Continued)

Comparison		adjusted p-value ≤ 0.05, fold change ≥ 2.0		
		Up		
	miRNA	Fold-change	Corrected p-value	Citation
PCMM vs. BMN	hsa-miR-21	4.0576706	0.01877952	(Xu, Brenn, Brown, Doherty and Melton, 2012)
	hsa-miR-3663-3p	2.369955	0.02128333	
	hsa-miR-4281	2.304322	0.04586014	
	hsa-miR-720	2.194011	0.01840767	
	hsa-miR-4286	2.009585	0.02708492	

Tab. 11-4: (Continued)

| Comparison | adjusted p-value ≤ 0.05, fold change ≥ 2.0 | | | |
| | | Down | | |
	miRNA	Fold-change	Corrected p-value	Citation
PCMM vs. BMN	hsa-miR-429	-104.78791	4.07E-09	(Xu, Brenn, Brown, Doherty and Melton, 2012)
	hsa-miR-204	-58.921413	0.02534578	(Yang and Wei, 2011)
	hsa-miR-200a	-47.417885	0.03062929	(Elson-Schwab, et al., 2010, Gaur, Jewell, Liang, Ridzon, Moore, Chen, Ambros and Israel, 2007)
	hsa-miR-455-5p	-37.06338	0.03062929	(Xu, Brenn, Brown, Doherty and Melton, 2012)
	hsa-miR-149	-28.625843	0.04712249	(Xu, Brenn, Brown, Doherty and Melton, 2012)
	hsa-miR-664	-20.59269	0.01800365	(Grignol, Fairchild, Zimmerer, Lesinski, Walker, Magro, Kacher, Karpa, Clark, Nuovo, Lehman, Volinia, Agnese, Croce and Carson, 2011)

Tab. 11-4: (Continued)

Comparison	miRNA	Fold-change	Corrected p-value	Citation
adjusted p-value ≤ 0.05, fold change ≥ 2.0				
Down				
PCMM vs. BMN	hsa-miR-183	-16.913725	0.02834839	(Xu, Brenn, Brown, Doherty and Melton, 2012)
	hsa-miR-24-1*	-13.069493	0.04712249	
	hsa-miR-574-3p	-2.9407115	0.04712249	(Jukic, Rao, Kelly, Skaf, Drogowski, Kirkwood and Panelli, 2010)
	hsa-miR-23b	-2.798827	0.04485515	(Philippidou, Schmitt, Moser, Margue, Nazarov, Muller, Vallar, Nashan, Behrmann and Kreis, 2010)
	hsa-miR-125b	-2.3373234	0.04712249	(Glud, Rossing, Hother, Holst, Hastrup, Nielsen, Gniadecki and Drzewiecki, 2010)
	hsa-let-7a	-2.0023308	0.01186657	(Muller and Bosserhoff, 2008)

Tab. 11-4: (Continued)

Comparison	miRNA	Fold-change	p-value	Citation
			p-value ≤ 0.05. fold-change ≥ 2.0	
			Up	
PCMM vs. CMMM	hsa-miR-31	26.18982	0.006390245	
	hsa-miR-486-5p	22.908329	0.047547758	
	hsa-miR-4291	22.49766	0.000993379	
	hsa-miR-31*	16.113304	0.007797695	
	hsa-miR-17*	10.482874	0.034202397	(Leidinger, Keller, Borries, Reichrath, Rass, Jager, Lenhof and Meese, 2010)
	hsa-miR-145*	5.8212833	0.026987018	
	hsa-miR-4317	4.8699017	0.044183668	
	hsa-miR-1	4.1045427	0.0363784	
	hsa-miR-92a	2.327539	0.017932193	(Levati, Alvino, Pagani, Arcelli, Caporaso, Bondanza, Di Leva, Ferracin, Volinia, Bonmassar, Croce and D'Atri, 2009)
SSM vs. NMM	hsa-miR-664*	21.752323	0.004301061	
	hsa-miR-766	8.938961	0.04847504	

Tab. 11-4: (Continued)

Comparison	miRNA	Fold-change	Down p-value	Citation
			p-value ≤ 0.05. fold-change ≥ 2.0	
PCMM vs. CMMM	hsa-miR-542-5p	-21.225138	0.022108719	
	hsa-miR-34c-5p	-15.023849	0.027650215	
	hsa-miR-424	-3.8762648	0.011773768	
	hsa-miR-148a	-2.3403358	0.0334941	
	hsa-miR-15b	-2.0360043	3.08E-06	(Satzger, Mattern, Kuettler, Weinspach, Voelker, Kapp and Gutzmer, 2010)
SSM vs. NMM			0	

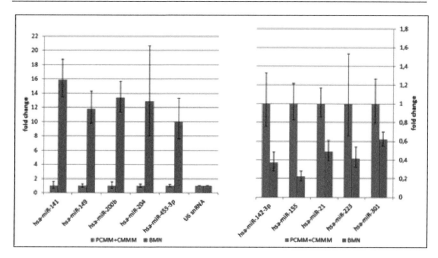

Fig. 11-3:   Results for differential expression in the comparison between benign melanocytic nevi (BMN) and the combined group of primary cutaneous malignant melanoma (PCMM) and cutaneous malignant melanoma metastasis (CMMM). Down-regulated miRNAs are displayed on the left side of the figure, and up-regulated miRNAs are displayed on the right side of the figure.

Hsa-miR-21 and hsa-miR-21*, which originate from the opposite arms of the same pre-miRNA were both differentially expressed in our study consistent with previous reports for these miRNAs in several forms of cancer (Meng, et al., 2007). Hsa-miR-21 is a known oncogene, as it has been shown to down-regulate the tumor suppressor gene programmed cell death 4 (PDCD4) in breast and colon cancers, as well as the tumor suppressor phosphatase and tensin homolog (PTEN) in human hepatocellular carcinoma (Asangani, et al., 2008, Frankel, et al., 2008). Hsa-miR-21 has been shown to regulate the metastatic behavior of melanoma cells by promoting cell proliferation, survival, and migration with increasing expression levels observed from dysplastic nevi to PCMM to CMMM (Jiang, et al., 2011, Yang, et al., 2011). Furthermore, hsa-miR-21 together with hsa-miR-155 has been associated with the modulation of mitotic activity and lesion depth of borderline melanocytic lesions (Grignol, et al., 2011). Hsa-miR-142-3p and hsa-miR-1280 are part of a characteristic miRNA expression profile, which was found in the blood cells of patients with cutaneous malignant melanoma (Leidinger, Keller, Borries, Reichrath, Rass, Jager, Lenhof and Meese, 2010). Hsa-miR-142-3p and hsa-miR-31 have been shown to be part of a miRNA signature that is associated with acral, but not non-acral, melanomas (Chan, et al., 2011). Hsa-miR-142-3p, hsa-miR-1280 and hsa-miR-31 were also differentially expressed in our group of samples. For a detailed list of the differentially expressed miRNAs, see Tab. 11-4.

In our study, we also observed several significantly downregulated miRNAs, which have been previously reported to be associated with CMM. Among the downregulated miRNAs is a member of the hsa-miR-29 family that has previously been found to down-regulate the DNA methyltransferases *DNMT3A* and *DNMT3B*, with *DNMT3B* playing a significant role in CMM progression and being an epigenetic CMM biomarker (Nguyen, et al., 2011). Although previously reported to be upregulated, hsa-miR-429 and hsa-miR-200a were downregulated in our study (Zhang, et al., 2006). We suspect that this discrepancy could be a cell culture-based phenomenon. As previously discussed by Molnár et al., healthy *in vitro* cultured melanocytes express a variety of known cell surface markers, whereas *in vivo*, melanocytes repress the expression of some of these genes when in a skin-like microenvironment (Molnar, Tamasi, Bakos, Wiener and Falus, 2008).

Therefore, one may assume that *in vitro* cultured melanocytes do not accurately reflect the *in vivo* changes in melanocyte miRNA expression, which may help explain the conflicting results among the currently available miRNA profiling studies (Molnar, Tamasi, Bakos, Wiener and Falus, 2008).

Hsa-miR-455-5p and hsa-miR-29c* have been shown to be downregulated in CMM in older adults (> 60 years) significantly more than in CMM in younger adults (Jukic, et al., 2010). Hsa-miR-204, which was shown to be down-regulated in this study was also reported to be significantly down-regulated in uveal melanomas compared to normal uveal tissues (Yang and Wei, 2011).

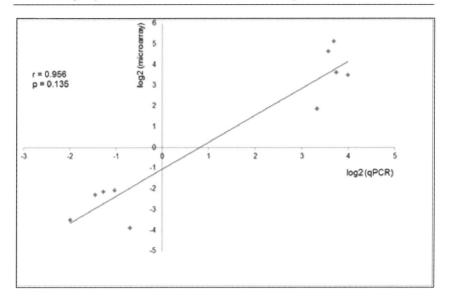

Fig. 11-4: A scatter plot based on the log2 qRT-PCR (qPCR) and microarray results of the different miRNAs in the comparison between benign melanocytic nevi (BMN) and the combined group of primary cutaneous malignant melanoma (PCMM) and cutaneous malignant melanoma metastasis (CMMM). Included in this plot are a linear trend line, as well as the r- and p-values in the upper left corner representing the correlation analysis. A high degree (r= 0.956) of correlation is observed between the qPCR and microarray results with no significant differences between the qPCR and microarray data (p-value=0.135).

Hsa-miR-149 has been reported to be up-regulated in cKit-negative melanoma cells that were isolated from tumors; however, our study shows a downregulation of hsa-miR-149 (Igoucheva and Alexeev, 2009). Another miRNA, hsa-miR-183 was downregulated in our study but was found to be upregulated in a previous study using melanoma cell lines (Zhang, Huang, Yang, Greshock, Megraw, Giannakakis, Liang, Naylor, Barchetti, Ward, Yao, Medina, O'Brien-Jenkins, Katsaros, Hatzigeorgiou, Gimotty, Weber and Coukos, 2006). We also report the downregulation of hsa-miR-664, although this miRNA has previously been reported to be upregulated in the blood samples of melanoma patients (Leidinger, Keller, Borries, Reichrath, Rass, Jager, Lenhof and Meese, 2010).

Members of the hsa-mir-200 family, hsa-mir-200a, b and c and hsa-miR-141 were all down-regulated in our study but were reported to be both up- and down-regulated in other miRNA expression studies based on melanoma cell lines (Elson-Schwab, et al., 2010, Gaur, et al., 2007). The hsa-mir-200 family has been shown to regulate the morphological plasticity of melanoma cells and tumor progression by suppressing the epithelial-mesenchymal transition, which is thought to be an early but necessary step in tumor metastasis (Elson-Schwab, Lorentzen and Marshall, 2010). The hedgehog signaling pathway, which is involved in the epithelial-mesenchymal transition, induces TGF-beta 1, which has been shown to mediate the downregulation of hsa-mir-200a, hsa-mir-200b and hsa-mir-200c (Katoh and Katoh, 2008). In a recent profiling study on paraffin-embedded melanoma samples, hsa-mir-200c was down-regulated, which is consistent with our study (Xu, et al., 2012).

Hsa-miR-224 and hsa-miR-224* were also downregulated in our study; however, hsa-miR-224 and hsa-miR-224 have been previously reported to be both up- and down-regulated melanoma cell lines (Elson-Schwab, Lorentzen and Marshall, 2010, Gaur, Jewell, Liang, Ridzon, Moore, Chen, Ambros and Israel, 2007).

Hsa-miR-192 was previously reported to be down-regulated in melanoma cell lines and was also down-regulated in the patient tumors included in our study (Caramuta, et al., 2010, Zhang, Huang, Yang, Greshock, Megraw, Giannakakis, Liang, Naylor, Barchetti, Ward, Yao, Medina, O'Brien-Jenkins, Katsaros, Hatzigeorgiou, Gimotty, Weber and Coukos, 2006). Hsa-miR-455-3p was also significantly downregulated in our study, which is also consistent with a previous study by Segura et al. in which they compared PCMM and CMMM tumors to BMN tumors (Segura, Belitskaya-Levy, Rose, Zakrzewski, Gaziel, Hanniford, Darvishian, Berman, Shapiro, Pavlick, Osman and Hernando, 2010). Hsa-miR-186, which down-regulates the expression of the pro-apoptotic purinergic P2X7 receptor, showed a decrease in expression in our study while it has been reported as significantly elevated in the blood samples of melanoma patients and in melanoma cell lines (Leidinger, Keller, Borries, Reichrath, Rass, Jager, Lenhof and Meese, 2010). Consistent with a previous report by Jukic et al., the group of PCMM and CMMM tumors in our study showed a down-regulation of hsa-miR-574-3p (Jukic, Rao, Kelly, Skaf, Drogowski, Kirkwood and Panelli, 2010). Philippidou et al. also described the downregulation of hsa-miR-23b in melanoma specimens, which was consistent with the observations in our group of patient tumors (Philippidou, Schmitt, Moser, Margue, Nazarov, Muller, Vallar, Nashan, Behrmann and Kreis, 2010). Hsa-miR-100 has also been reported to be downregulated in melanoma cell lines, and hsa-miR-125b has been reported to be downregulated in PCMM samples (Glud, et al., 2010, Zhang, Huang, Yang, Greshock, Megraw, Giannakakis, Liang, Naylor, Barchetti, Ward, Yao, Medina, O'Brien-Jenkins, Katsaros, Hatzigeorgiou, Gimotty, Weber and Coukos, 2006). The highly conserved members of the let-7 family, such as hsa-let-7a are non-coding tumor suppressor genes previously shown to be downregulated in CMM and shown to have an impact on the invasive potential of melanoma cells (Muller and Bosserhoff, 2008).

Collectively, our results strongly suggest the confirmation of numerous miRNAs that have been previously reported to be differentially expressed in cutaneous malignant melanomas. However, our results also describe several previously unidentified differentially expressed miRNA candidates that warrant further investigation in larger studies to confirm our preliminary microarray results. These studies will be useful in the detailed evaluation of these miRNAs at a functional level and will serve as a potential starting point to evaluate the significance of these miRNAs in diagnostic, prognostic and therapeutic applications.

11.5 Conclusion

The current study was performed to find miRNA candidates previously not linked to PCMM or CMMM formation based on miRBase version 16. In this report, we have described a preliminary list of miRNA candidates that have not previously been linked to cutaneous malignant melanoma and warrant further validation and functional analysis.

11.6 Acknowledgements

This work was generously supported in part by Fleur Hiege Stiftung gegen Hautkrebs in Hamburg, Germany. The financial sponsors had no role in the study design, data collection and analysis, decision to publish, or preparation of the manuscript. The authors are grateful to Dr. Cornelia Graf and Stefan Kotschote, MS for technical advice.

11.7 References

Ambros V (2004) The functions of animal microRNAs. Nature 431:350-355

Asangani IA, Rasheed SA, Nikolova DA, Leupold JH, Colburn NH, Post S, Allgayer H (2008) MicroRNA-21 (miR-21) post-transcriptionally downregulates tumor suppressor Pdcd4 and stimulates invasion, intravasation and metastasis in colorectal cancer. Oncogene 27:2128-2136

Bartel DP (2004) MicroRNAs: genomics, biogenesis, mechanism, and function. Cell 116:281-297

Benjamini Y, Hochberg Y (1995) Controlling the false discovery rate: a practical and powerful approach to multiple testing. J R Stat Soc Ser B 57:289-300

Bonazzi VF, Irwin D, Hayward NK (2009) Identification of candidate tumor suppressor genes inactivated by promoter methylation in melanoma. Genes Chromosomes Cancer 48:10-21

Bonazzi VF, Stark MS, Hayward NK (2011) MicroRNA regulation of melanoma progression. Melanoma Res

Boone B, Jacobs K, Ferdinande L, Taildeman J, Lambert J, Peeters M, Bracke M, Pauwels P, Brochez L (2011) EGFR in melanoma: clinical significance and potential therapeutic target. J Cutan Pathol 38:492-502

Busse A, Keilholz U (2011) Role of TGF-beta in Melanoma. Curr Pharm Biotechnol

Caramuta S, Egyhazi S, Rodolfo M, Witten D, Hansson J, Larsson C, Lui WO (2010) MicroRNA expression profiles associated with mutational status and survival in malignant melanoma. J Invest Dermatol 130:2062-2070

Chan E, Patel R, Nallur S, Ratner E, Bacchiocchi A, Hoyt K, Szpakowski S, Godshalk S, Ariyan S, Sznol M, Halaban R, Krauthammer M, Tuck D, Slack FJ, Weidhaas JB (2011) MicroRNA signatures differentiate melanoma subtypes. Cell Cycle 10:1845-1852

de Wit PE, Moretti S, Koenders PG, Weterman MA, van Muijen GN, Gianotti B, Ruiter DJ (1992) Increasing epidermal growth factor receptor expression in human melanocytic tumor progression. J Invest Dermatol 99:168-173

Edgar R, Domrachev M, Lash AE (2002) Gene Expression Omnibus: NCBI gene expression and hybridization array data repository. Nucleic Acids Res 30:207-210

Elson-Schwab I, Lorentzen A, Marshall CJ (2010) MicroRNA-200 family members differentially regulate morphological plasticity and mode of melanoma cell invasion. PLoS One 5:

Fan T, Jiang S, Chung N, Alikhan A, Ni C, Lee CC, Hornyak TJ (2011) EZH2-dependent suppression of a cellular senescence phenotype in melanoma cells by inhibition of p21/CDKN1A expression. Mol Cancer Res 9:418-429

Faraoni I, Antonetti FR, Cardone J, Bonmassar E (2009) miR-155 gene: a typical multifunctional microRNA. Biochim Biophys Acta 1792:497-505

Frankel LB, Christoffersen NR, Jacobsen A, Lindow M, Krogh A, Lund AH (2008) Programmed cell death 4 (PDCD4) is an important functional target of the microRNA miR-21 in breast cancer cells. J Biol Chem 283:1026-1033

Friedman RC, Farh KK, Burge CB, Bartel DP (2009) Most mammalian mRNAs are conserved targets of microRNAs. Genome Res 19:92-105

Gaur A, Jewell DA, Liang Y, Ridzon D, Moore JH, Chen C, Ambros VR, Israel MA (2007) Characterization of microRNA expression levels and their biological correlates in human cancer cell lines. Cancer Res 67:2456-2468

Geraldo MV, Yamashita AS, Kimura ET (2011) MicroRNA miR-146b-5p regulates signal transduction of TGF-beta by repressing SMAD4 in thyroid cancer. Oncogene

Glud M, Rossing M, Hother C, Holst L, Hastrup N, Nielsen FC, Gniadecki R, Drzewiecki KT (2010) Downregulation of miR-125b in metastatic cutaneous malignant melanoma. Melanoma Res 20:479-484

Grignol V, Fairchild ET, Zimmerer JM, Lesinski GB, Walker MJ, Magro CM, Kacher JE, Karpa VI, Clark J, Nuovo G, Lehman A, Volinia S, Agnese DM, Croce CM, Carson WE, 3rd (2011) miR-21 and miR-155 are associated with mitotic activity and lesion depth of borderline melanocytic lesions. Br J Cancer 105:1023-1029

Howell PM, Jr., Li X, Riker AI, Xi Y (2010) MicroRNA in Melanoma. Ochsner J 10:83-92

Igoucheva O, Alexeev V (2009) MicroRNA-dependent regulation of cKit in cutaneous melanoma. Biochem Biophys Res Commun 379:790-794

Jiang L, Lv X, Li J, Li X, Li W, Li Y (2011) The status of microRNA-21 expression and its clinical significance in human cutaneous malignant melanoma. Acta Histochem

Jiang Q, Wang Y, Hao Y, Juan L, Teng M, Zhang X, Li M, Wang G, Liu Y (2009) miR2Disease: a manually curated database for microRNA deregulation in human disease. Nucleic Acids Res 37:D98-104

Jukic DM, Rao UN, Kelly L, Skaf JS, Drogowski LM, Kirkwood JM, Panelli MC (2010) Microrna profiling analysis of differences between the melanoma of young adults and older adults. J Transl Med 8:27

Karube Y, Tanaka H, Osada H, Tomida S, Tatematsu Y, Yanagisawa K, Yatabe Y, Takamizawa J, Miyoshi S, Mitsudomi T, Takahashi T (2005) Reduced expression of Dicer associated with poor prognosis in lung cancer patients. Cancer Sci 96:111-115

Katakowski M, Zheng X, Jiang F, Rogers T, Szalad A, Chopp M (2010) MiR-146b-5p suppresses EGFR expression and reduces in vitro migration and invasion of glioma. Cancer Invest 28:1024-1030

Katoh Y, Katoh M (2008) Hedgehog signaling, epithelial-to-mesenchymal transition and miRNA (review). Int J Mol Med 22:271-275

Lee YS, Kim HK, Chung S, Kim KS, Dutta A (2005) Depletion of human micro-RNA miR-125b reveals that it is critical for the proliferation of differentiated cells but not for the down-regulation of putative targets during differentiation. J Biol Chem 280:16635-16641

Leidinger P, Keller A, Borries A, Reichrath J, Rass K, Jager SU, Lenhof HP, Meese E (2010) High-throughput miRNA profiling of human melanoma blood samples. BMC Cancer 10:262

Lesinski GB, Raig ET, Zimmerer JM, Karpa V, Nuovo G, Lehman A, Peters S, Kacher JE, Magro CM, Croce CM, Carson WE (2008) Micro-RNA-21 and micro-RNA-155 as predictors of a malignant phenotype in melanocytic lesions. J Clin Oncol 26:9001

Levati L, Alvino E, Pagani E, Arcelli D, Caporaso P, Bondanza S, Di Leva G, Ferracin M, Volinia S, Bonmassar E, Croce CM, D'Atri S (2009) Altered expression of selected microRNAs in melanoma: antiproliferative and proapoptotic activity of miRNA-155. Int J Oncol 35:393-400

Lewis BP, Burge CB, Bartel DP (2005) Conserved seed pairing, often flanked by adenosines, indicates that thousands of human genes are microRNA targets. Cell 120:15-20

Lu Z, Li Y, Takwi A, Li B, Zhang J, Conklin DJ, Young KH, Martin R (2011) miR-301a as an NF-kappaB activator in pancreatic cancer cells. EMBO J 30:57-67

McHugh JB, Fullen DR, Ma L, Kleer CG, Su LD (2007) Expression of polycomb group protein EZH2 in nevi and melanoma. J Cutan Pathol 34:597-600

Meng F, Henson R, Wehbe-Janek H, Ghoshal K, Jacob ST, Patel T (2007) MicroRNA-21 regulates expression of the PTEN tumor suppressor gene in human hepatocellular cancer. Gastroenterology 133:647-658

miRBase (2011).

Molnar V, Tamasi V, Bakos B, Wiener Z, Falus A (2008) Changes in miRNA expression in solid tumors: an miRNA profiling in melanomas. Semin Cancer Biol 18:111-122

Mueller DW, Bosserhoff AK (2009) Role of miRNAs in the progression of malignant melanoma. Br J Cancer 101:551-556

Mueller DW, Bosserhoff AK (2011) miRNAs in Malignant Melanoma. In: Bosserhoff AK (ed) Melanoma Development: Molecular Biology. Springer, New York, pp 121

Mueller DW, Rehli M, Bosserhoff AK (2009) miRNA expression profiling in melanocytes and melanoma cell lines reveals miRNAs associated with formation and progression of malignant melanoma. J Invest Dermatol 129:1740-1751

Muller DW, Bosserhoff AK (2008) Integrin beta 3 expression is regulated by let-7a miRNA in malignant melanoma. Oncogene 27:6698-6706

Nguyen T, Kuo C, Nicholl MB, Sim MS, Turner RR, Morton DL, Hoon DS (2011) Downregulation of microRNA-29c is associated with hypermethylation of tumor-related genes and disease outcome in cutaneous melanoma. Epigenetics 6:388-394

Philippidou D, Schmitt M, Moser D, Margue C, Nazarov PV, Muller A, Vallar L, Nashan D, Behrmann I, Kreis S (2010) Signatures of microRNAs and selected microRNA target genes in human melanoma. Cancer Res 70:4163-4173

Quackenbush J (2001) Computational analysis of microarray data. Nat Rev Genet 2:418-427

Sand M, Gambichler T, Sand D, Altmeyer P, Stuecker M, Bechara FG (2011) Immunohistochemical expression patterns of the microRNA-processing enzyme Dicer in cutaneous malignant melanomas, benign melanocytic nevi and dysplastic melanocytic nevi. Eur J Dermatol 21:18-21

Sand M, Gambichler T, Sand D, Skrygan M, Altmeyer P, Bechara FG (2009) MicroRNAs and the skin: tiny players in the body's largest organ. J Dermatol Sci 53:169-175

Sand M, Skrygan M, Georgas D, Sand D, Gambichler T, Altmeyer P, Bechara FG (2012) The miRNA machinery in primary cutaneous malignant melanoma, cutaneous malignant melanoma metastases and benign melanocytic nevi. Cell Tissue Res

Sander S, Bullinger L, Klapproth K, Fiedler K, Kestler HA, Barth TF, Moller P, Stilgenbauer S, Pollack JR, Wirth T (2008) MYC stimulates EZH2 expression by repression of its negative regulator miR-26a. Blood 112:4202-4212

Satzger I, Mattern A, Kuettler U, Weinspach D, Voelker B, Kapp A, Gutzmer R (2010) MicroRNA-15b represents an independent prognostic parameter and is correlated with tumor cell proliferation and apoptosis in malignant melanoma. Int J Cancer 126:2553-2562

Schultz J, Lorenz P, Gross G, Ibrahim S, Kunz M (2008) MicroRNA let-7b targets important cell cycle molecules in malignant melanoma cells and interferes with anchorage-independent growth. Cell Res 18:549-557

Segura MF, Belitskaya-Levy I, Rose AE, Zakrzewski J, Gaziel A, Hanniford D, Darvishian F, Berman RS, Shapiro RL, Pavlick AC, Osman I, Hernando E (2010) Melanoma MicroRNA signature predicts post-recurrence survival. Clin Cancer Res 16:1577-1586

Sheng Y, Engstrom PG, Lenhard B (2007) Mammalian microrna prediction through a support vector machine model of sequence and structure. PLoS One 2:e946

Sigalotti L, Covre A, Fratta E, Parisi G, Colizzi F, Rizzo A, Danielli R, Nicolay HJ, Coral S, Maio M (2010) Epigenetics of human cutaneous melanoma: setting the stage for new therapeutic strategies. J Transl Med 8:56

Sokal R, Michener C (1958) A statistical method for evaluating systematic relationships. . University of Kansas Science Bulletin 38:1409-1438

Takamizawa J, Konishi H, Yanagisawa K, Tomida S, Osada H, Endoh H, Harano T, Yatabe Y, Nagino M, Nimura Y, Mitsudomi T, Takahashi T (2004) Reduced expression of the let-7 microRNAs in human lung cancers in association with shortened postoperative survival. Cancer Res 64:3753-3756

Thompson KL, Pine PS, Rosenzweig BA, Turpaz Y, Retief J (2007) Characterization of the effect of sample quality on high density oligonucleotide microarray data using progressively degraded rat liver RNA. BMC Biotechnol 7:57

Ueda Y, Richmond A (2006) NF-kappaB activation in melanoma. Pigment Cell Res 19:112-124

Xu Y, Brenn T, Brown ER, Doherty V, Melton DW (2012) Differential expression of microRNAs during melanoma progression: miR-200c, miR-205 and miR-211 are downregulated in melanoma and act as tumour suppressors. Br J Cancer

Yang C, Wei W (2011) The miRNA expression profile of the uveal melanoma. Sci China Life Sci 54:351-358

Yang CH, Yue J, Pfeffer SR, Handorf CR, Pfeffer LM (2011) MicroRNA miR-21 regulates the metastatic behavior of B16 melanoma cells. J Biol Chem 286:39172-39178

Yeung ML, Yasunaga J, Bennasser Y, Dusetti N, Harris D, Ahmad N, Matsuoka M, Jeang KT (2008) Roles for microRNAs, miR-93 and miR-130b, and tumor protein 53-induced nuclear protein 1 tumor suppressor in cell growth dysregulation by human T-cell lymphotrophic virus 1. Cancer Res 68:8976-8985

Zhang JD, Biczok R, Ruschhaupt M (2011) The ddCt Algorithm for the Analysis of Quantitative Real-Time PCR (qRT-PCR).

Zhang L, Huang J, Yang N, Greshock J, Megraw MS, Giannakakis A, Liang S, Naylor TL, Barchetti A, Ward MR, Yao G, Medina A, O'Brien-Jenkins A, Katsaros D, Hatzigeorgiou A, Gimotty PA, Weber BL, Coukos G (2006) microRNAs exhibit high frequency genomic alterations in human cancer. Proc Natl Acad Sci U S A 103:9136-9141

Zhang Z, Sun H, Dai H, Walsh RM, Imakura M, Schelter J, Burchard J, Dai X, Chang AN, Diaz RL, Marszalek JR, Bartz SR, Carleton M, Cleary MA, Linsley PS, Grandori C (2009) MicroRNA miR-210 modulates cellular response to hypoxia through the MYC antagonist MNT. Cell Cycle 8:2756-2768

12 Paper 8: MicroRNAs and the skin: tiny players in the body's largest organ[*]

12.1 Introduction

Humans inherit 23 chromosomes from each parent to form a diploid genome consisting of 46 chromosomes. Although the exact number of total protein-coding genes within our genome remains unclear, initial estimates of >100,000 genes have recently been refined to 20,000-25,000 genes [1]. However, only a small subset of these genes is actually active, giving rise to approximately 210 different cell types and tissues of the human body, including the skin. While much focus and research has been devoted to protein-coding genes, the majority of the genome actually consists of non-coding genes and regions. For a long time, these non-coding DNA regions were regarded as evolutionarily conserved junk DNA. Recent findings, however, proved this to be vastly untrue. The majority of the DNA in our genomes, initially labeled as unnecessary and useless, is actively transcribed into functional primary RNA transcripts or non-coding RNAs (ncRNAs). At the time, only a select few ncRNAs were characterized, namely, ribosomal RNAs (rRNAs) and transfer RNAs (tRNAs), which are important for the translation machinery. The significance of other ncRNAs only became clear when RNA silencing mechanisms were discovered. In the past decade, significant research in eukaryotic cells showed that ncRNAs play an immensely important role in the post-transcriptional regulation of up to 30% of all our genes. This post-transcriptional regulation is mainly accomplished by two types of ncRNAs, small interfering RNAs (siRNAs) and microRNAs (miRNAs).

Although miRNA research in the field of dermatology is still relatively new, miRNAs have been the subject of much dermatological interest. Some intriguing results have been achieved in this rapidly developing field, which is the focus of this review.

---

[*] Co-authors: Thilo Gambichler, Daniel Sand, Marina Skrygan, Peter Altmeyer, Falk G. Bechara

12.2   RNA interference and microRNA discovery

In 1990, a phenomenon called gene or RNA silencing was first described in widely cultivated flowering plants. Basically, when a cloned gene was incorporated into the genome of the petunia plant, not only did it produce a stimulating effect on the purple pigment gene, but it also inhibited expression of homologous sequences. This intriguing phenomenon was aptly named homology-dependent gene silencing [2].

Shortly thereafter in 1998, Fire et al. [3] described a similar post-transcriptional gene silencing mechanism in the nematode *Caenorhabditis elegans* (*C. elegans*) called RNA interference (RNAi). Both Fire and Mello subsequently received the Nobel Prize for Physiology and Medicine in 2006 for their pioneering work. In brief, they injected single-stranded sense and antisense RNA as well as double-stranded RNA (dsRNA) into the *C. elegans* worm and tested for a phenotypic effect. They observed that injection of dsRNA led to an expected full loss of the target mRNA expression in the worm, while injection of single-stranded RNA (regardless whether it was sense or antisense) led to no or very weak loss of target mRNA expression. Thus, physiological gene silencing, which was only known in plants at the time, was also demonstrated in worms. They concluded that the presence of dsRNA led to a loss of target mRNA and a consequent change in phenotype. However, it was unclear if the observed gene silencing was acting through a transcriptional or post-transcriptional mechanism. That same year, Montgomery et al. [4] shed some light on this question and showed that the dsRNA exerted its effect at the post-transcriptional level. RNAi was also demonstrated to occur in a variety of other organisms such as fruit flies, plants and zebrafish. In cultured mammalian cells, however, the RNAi silencing response occurred only when exposed to short (21 nucleotides) dsRNAs [5], which were later identified as small interfering RNAs (siRNAs) that acted by blocking expression of a target mRNA *in vivo* [6]. In the cell, the long dsRNA was actually cut into smaller pieces of 21-25 nucleotides (nt) in length and inhibited specific mRNAs through basepairing. This endogenous small RNA was named microRNA and represents one of the most important components of RNAi-mediated gene silencing. The first miRNA, named lin-4, was discovered by Victor Ambros and colleagues back in 1993 [7]. While performing a genetic screen in the *C. elegans* worm they found a 22-nucleotide long small RNA molecule, which was involved in developmental timing. Seven years later the second miRNA described was let-7, currently called let-7a by Reinhart et al in 2000 [8]. In 2001 Grishok et al. demonstrated that inactivation of genes related to RNAi pathway genes such as a homolog of Drosophila Dicer (dcr-1) and two homologs of rde-1 (alg-1 and alg-2) caused heterochronic phenotypes similar to lin-4 and let-7 mutations [9]. They showed that dcr-1, alg-1 and alg-2 are necessary for the maturation and activity of both lin-4 and let-7. The RNAi mechanisms described by Fire et al. were linked to the mechanism of action by which miRNAs function. Both siRNA and miRNA share some characteristics (20-25 nt length, 5´-phosphate, and 3`-hydroxyl) and cannot be distinguished on the basis of their function. They can each cleave complementary mRNA targets and decrease the expression of partially complementary targets. However, there are some important differences. The regulatory activity of siRNA is restricted as it binds via complementary Watson-Crick base pairing within the exons of mRNA. In contrast, miRNA binds via base paring with partially complementary sequences present in the 3´UTRs of target transcripts. However the most important difference is the fact that siRNA is not solely an endogenous biological molecule. Some siRNAs are synthetic molecules and the result of exogenously introduced transgenes, viruses or rouge genetic elements. Although rare in mammals, there are also biological siRNAs which come from long endogenous dsRNA molecules [10]. In contrast miRNA is solely endogenously encoded in the genome, and represents a heritable as well as a stable post-transcriptional regulatory mechanism that controls a variety of cellular activities. Since its discovery, miRNAs have received considerable interest in basic research, enabling for the discovery and treatment of a variety of diseases.

12.3 miRNA biogenesis

MicroRNAs are small 21-25 nt RNA molecules that are essential regulators of a wide range of cellular processes. miRNAs play a key role in regulating gene expression by both promoting mRNA degradation and inhibiting mRNA translation, with an emphasis on the latter in mammals [11]. For the expression of miRNA three different transcriptional regulatory mechanisms have been described. Intronic miRNAs are encoded in the gene transcript precursors and share the same promoter with the encoded gene transcripts. They require type-II RNA polymerases (Pol-II) and spliceosomal components for their biogenesis. Intergenic miRNAs are located in the non-coding regions and transcribed by unidentified promoters [12]. The third group is called polycistronic miRNAs which are derived from primary transcripts containing multiple hairpins, with different hairpins giving rise to different miRNAs [10]. The biogenesis of miRNAs is complex and includes several steps. Similar to protein-coding genes, miRNAs are transcribed by RNA polymerase II in mammalian cells (Fig 12-1). The primary miRNA transcript (pri-miRNA) is usually several kilobases long, poladenylated at its 3′ end and capped with a 7-methylguanosine cap at its 5' end [13]. The intranuclear RNase III enzyme Drosha then cleaves the pri-miRNA, which may contain multiple miRNA hairpins, into several precursor miRNAs (pre-miRNAs) [14]. The cofactor DGCR8 (DiGeorge syndrome critical region gene 8/Pasha) is essential for Drosha activity and is thought to initiate pri-miRNA binding, as it contains two dsRNA-binding domains [15,16]. Both Drosha and its cofactor DGCR8/Pasha constitute the microprocessor complex, which then cuts the pri-miRNA at the ssRNA/dsRNA junction located at the base of the pri-miRNA hairpins. The cut is about one dsRNA helical turn in length and leaves a small 3' overhang [15]. The resulting pre-miRNAs are 70-90 nt long and have characteristic stem-loop hairpin secondary structures. The pre-miRNA also contains a 2 nt overhang at its 3′ end, which is bound by exportin 5 in the presence of its cofactor, Ran-guanine triphosphatase (Ran-GTP) [17]. Exportin 5 belongs to the karyopherin family of nucleocytoplasmic transport factors and exports cargo for the pre-miRNA [18]. Exportin 5 is also responsible for the nucleocytoplasmic transport of viral hairpin RNAs and some tRNAs. Once the pre-miRNA has been exported into the cytoplasm, a second RNase III enzyme called Dicer processes the pre-miRNA with the help of several cofactors (TAR RNA-Binding Protein or TRBP and

PACT). Dicer cuts the pre-miRNA at a predetermined distance from the 3´ end, resulting in short fragments ranging from 21 to 27 nt in length with a 2 nt overhang at its 3´ end [19]. Processing by Dicer results in a mature miRNA strand and an opposing strand (marked as miRNA*), which is degraded. The miRNA is now ready to be incorporated into the RNA-induced silencing complex (RISC).

12.4 miRNA function

The 3´ end of the mature miRNA is loaded into RISC with the help of an Argonaute protein and is now capable of modulating gene expression [20]. The integrated miRNA guides RISC to its specific mRNA target through basepair complementarity, and RISC anneals to the target mRNA to disrupt translation. Depending on the degree of complementarity between the miRNA and target mRNA, two different mechanisms of RISC-mediated gene regulation occur. In the case of nearly complete complementarity, RISC cleaves the target mRNA [21], thus preventing its translation. In the case of limited complementarity, translation is suppressed by mRNA decapping and/or deadenylation [8]. Thus far, 695 different human miRNAs have been described, predicted to control approximately 30% of all genes in the genome [22]. Some of the miRNAs have been linked to the pathogenesis of a variety of cutaneous disorders, which are briefly reviewed as follows.

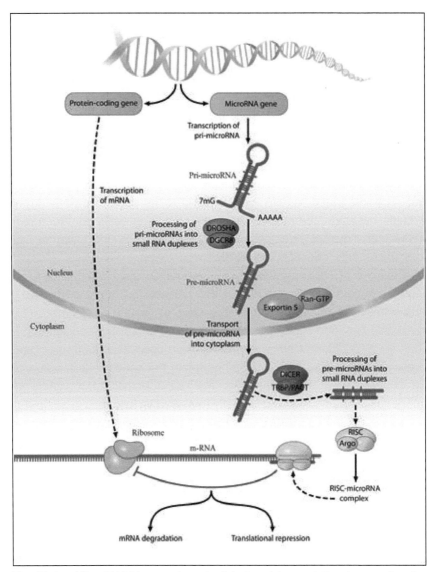

Fig. 12-1: MicroRNA biogenesis and related post-transcriptional gene silencing mechanisms (modified according to Chen) [63].

12.5   miRNAs and skin morphogenesis

Skin represents the largest organ in the human body, and its morphogenesis has been shown to require highly coordinated and undisrupted miRNA metabolism. Yi et al. [23] have shown that high expression of several miRNAs in the epidermis and hair follicles is necessary for normal skin development. Using a mouse model of embryonic skin, progenitor cells were targeted for Dicer knockout – a pivotal enzyme involved in miRNA biogenesis. The skin epithelium in Dicer knockout mice failed to produce mature miRNAs, and embryonic hair germs were found to evaginate into the epidermis rather than invaginate normally toward the dermis. Expression of key signaling molecules involved in follicular proliferation, sonic hedgehog (Shh) and Notch homolog 1 (Notch1), was lost by postnatal day 7 [24]. Further investigation also revealed a disturbance in the architecture of other epithelial tissues including the filiform papillae of the tongue epithelium and rudimentary sweat glands of the plantar footpad epithelium. These results indicate that miRNAs are also necessary for the morphogenesis of other stratified epithelia.

The skin-specific miR-203 was recently linked to skin morphogenesis. Between embryonic day 13.5 to 15.5, miR-203 levels in mouse suprabasal cells showed a 25-fold increase in expression compared to that in basal cells. miR-203 represses p63 expression, an important factor in epidermal cell proliferation and differentiation [25]. P63 initiates epithelial stratification during embryogenesis and maintains the proliferative potential of mature keratinocytes in the basal layers of mature epidermis [26]. When undifferentiated stem cells begin to differentiate into stratified epithelium to build a protective skin barrier, miR-203 expression increases to suppress p63 activity. Downregulation of p63 then enables terminal differentiation to take place. miR-203 translationally represses p63, resulting in inhibition of the proliferative potential of epidermal stem cells [26]. However there is some debate concerning p63 and its role in stem cell biology and the question whether miR-203 is expressed in stem cells [27]. Further studies on this issue are needed.   Nevertheless, as high p63 expression was found in cancer cells, it will be of considerable interest to determine whether low miR-203 levels are associated with epithelial skin cancers.

12.6 miRNAs and skin cancer

As previously described, miRNAs and their key regulators are essential for morphogenesis of the skin and hair follicles. It is thus expected that a disruption of miRNA expression can be observed in various malignant skin lesions.

Melanoma is the most aggressive type of skin cancer, and it is resistant to therapy in its advanced stages. Thus far, melanoma and Kaposi's sarcoma are the only types of skin cancers that have been studied with regard to the role of miRNAs in disease pathogenesis [28].

Tab. 12-1: MicroRNAs which have been studied in cutaneous biology

MicroRNA	Function	Studies
let-7b	repressing expression of melanoma-promoting molecules such as cyclin D1, D3, Cdk4 and cyclin A in primary malignant melanomas	Schultz et al. [37]
miR-k12-11	viral microRNA (Kaposi Sarcoma Herpes Virus) which shares targets and binding sites (transcriptional regulators BACH-1, FOS and the proapoptotic effector LDOC-1) with human miR155; potentially involved in tumorigenesis	Skalsky et al. [40] Gottwein et al. [41]
miR-24	miR24 transcription is repressed by TGF-beta1, a modulator of fibroblastic mitosis during wound healing	Sun et al. [54]
miR-96	down–regulated in melanoma cell lines	Gaur et al. [30]
miR-125b	down-regulated in psoriasis, involved in post-transcriptional repression of TNF-α	Sonkoly et al. [46]
miR-137	modulating the expression of microphthalmia-associated transcription factor (MITF, a major regulator of melanocyte growth, maturation, apoptosis and pigmentation)	Bemis et al. [31]

Tab. 12-1: (Continued)

MicroRNA	Function	Studies
miR-146	up-regulated in melanoma cell lines	Gaur et al. [30]
miR-182	down–regulated in melanoma cell lines	Gaur et al. [30]
miR-183	down–regulated in melanoma cell lines	Gaur et al. [30]
miR-192	down–regulated in melanoma cell lines	Gaur et al. [30]
miR-194	down–regulated in melanoma cell lines	Gaur et al. [30]
miR-200a	down–regulated in melanoma cell lines	Gaur et al. [30]
miR-200bN	down–regulated in melanoma cell lines	Gaur et al. [30]
miR-200c	down–regulated in melanoma cell lines	Gaur et al. [30]
miR-203	down–regulated in melanoma cell lines	Gaur et al. [30]
miR-204	up-regulated in melanoma cell lines	Gaur et al. [30]
miR-211	up-regulated in melanoma cell lines	Gaur et al. [30]
miR-218-1	tumor suppressor located within the tumor suppressor gene SLIT2, 15 of 45 investigated primary melanoma cell lines showed copy number losses	Zhang et al. [29]
miR-221	controlling melanoma progression through downregulation of cyclin-dependent kinase inhibitor 1b (p27Kip1/CDKN1B) and c-KIT receptor	Felicetti et al. [34]
miR-222	"	Felicetti et al. [34]
miR-224	down–regulated in melanoma cell lines	Gaur et al. [30]
miR-335	down–regulated in melanoma cell lines	Gaur et al. [30]
miR-376	up-regulated in melanoma cell lines	Gaur et al. [30]

In 2006, Zhang et al. were the first to demonstrate the presence of high frequency copy abnormalities (gains and losses) in Dicer,

Argonaute2 and various miRNAs in primary cultured melanoma cell lines [29].

miR-218-1 is a tumor suppressor inactivated in breast, lung and colorectal cancers. It is located within the tumor suppressor gene SLIT2 (human homologue of *Drosophila Slit2*). In a study by Zhang et al. copy number losses of the region containing miR-218-1 and SLIT2 where shown in 33.3% of all investigated melanoma lines, thus indicating that miRNA copy number losses can occur simultaneously with inactivation of tumor suppressor genes [29].

In a genomic analysis of 241 miRNAs in eight melanoma lines, four miRNAs were found to be upregulated, and eleven were found to be downregulated [30]. Details of the latter analysis and other miRNA that have been identified or studied with respect to cutaneous biology are summarized in Table 12-1. Furthermore, miR-137 was shown to modulate expression of microphthalmia-associated transcription factor (MITF), which is a major regulator of melanocyte growth, maturation, apoptosis and pigmentation [31]. Ultraviolet radiation-induced sun tanning occurs through keratinocyte expression of α-melanocyte stimulating hormone (α-MSH), which then leads to melanocyte MITF expression. MITF induction is believed to protect the skin from DNA damage [32]. Additionally, expression of melanoma inhibitor of apoptosis (ML-IAP) in melanoma cells was recently shown to be MITF-dependent [33]. ML-IAP is a potent inhibitor of apoptosis and highly expressed in melanomas, and it likely contributes to chemotherapy resistance. Other miRNAs linked to melanoma progression are miR-221 and miR-222, which both indirectly regulate MITF expression [34]. miR-221 and miR-222 primarily control melanoma progression through downregulation of cyclin-dependent kinase inhibitor 1b (p27Kip1/CDKN1B) and c-KIT receptor, both of which play critical roles in melanocyte physiology and favor induction of malignant phenotypes [35]. Promyelocytic leukemia zinc finger (PLZF) is a tumor suppressor downregulated in many melanomas and has been identified as a transcriptional inhibitor of miR-221 and miR-222 [35,36]. *Let-7*, the founding member of the miRNA family, is also downregulated in melanomas compared to benign nevi [37]. Interestingly, *let-7* was the second miRNA (after *lin-4*) discovered in *C. elegans* to regulate developmental timing [8]. *Let-7* plays a role in melanoma development and progression, as its predicted targets include a series of cancer-promoting molecules, such as N-Ras, Raf, c-myc, cyclins D1 / D3 and cyclin-dependent kinase (Cdk) 4. Overexpression of *let-7b* results in inhibition of cell cycle progression and repressed expression of tumor-promoting molecules such as cyclin D1, D3, Cdk4 and cyclin A [37]. Let-7b and miR-199a together allow for significant discrimination between low and high metastatic risk for uveal melanoma; high expression of let-7b and miR-199a confers a high metastatic potential [38].

As discussed by Molnár et al., future miRNA research in melanoma must address two major issues [39]. The first is to obtain an unbiased representation of miRNA expression, as initial tumor samples may be contaminated with non-tumor cells. To circumvent this problem, laser-dissected samples are preferred to limit the degree of contamination with non-malignant cells. Secondly, healthy *in vitro* cultured melanocytes are often used as a control, as they express a variety of known cell surface markers. In contrast, melanocytes *in vivo* switch certain genes off when in a skin-like microenvironment. Thus, *in vitro* cultured melanocytes likely do not recapitulate *in vivo* melanocyte changes in miRNA expression.

Nevertheless, new approaches may guide researchers to better understand the formation of melanoma with the hope of possible future therapies.

Kaposi's sarcoma, a form of skin cancer associated with herpes virus (KSHV), has been identified as the causative agent of several diseases such as primary effusion lymphoma (PEL) and Castleman's disease. KSHV is a large DNA virus encoding over 80 different viral proteins and 12 different miRNAs, including miR-k12-11. Until recently no viral miRNAs have been reported to bind to mRNA targets via sites utilized by host miRNAs. Recently, human miR-155 was shown to share several targets and binding sites such as the transcriptional regulators BACH-1, FOS and the proapoptotic effector LDOC-1 with viral miR-k12-11 (40,41). It regulates the latter transcripts via the same binding sites utilized by the human miR-155. Mir-155 is part of the noncoding RNA of the B cell integration complex (BIC) gene which has been a suspected proto-oncogene in avian leukosis virus (ALV)- induced lymphomas and an enhancer of lymphomagenesis (42). The possibility that mir-k12-11 may play a role in tumorgenesis by interfering in the network of transcripts that are regulated by miR155 indicates a possible link between viral and non-viral tumorigenesis [28].

12.7 miRNAs and psoriasis

Psoriasis is a common chronic inflammatory skin condition characterized by accelerated keratinocyte proliferation, reduced apoptosis and epidermal infiltration of inflammatory cells that leads to the formation of skin plaques. Tumor necrosis factor (TNF)-α is a proinflammatory cytokine shown to play an important role in the pathogenesis of psoriasis [43].

Three different miRNAs have thus far been associated with this skin disease and linked to both innate immune responses and the TNF-α pathway [44]. miR-203 was the first miRNA found to be significantly overexpressed in psoriasis patients [45]. Upregulation of miR-203 leads to downregulation of suppressor of cytokine signaling-3 (SOCS-3) expression in psoriatic skin. SOCS-3 is an inhibitor of the signal transducer and activator of transcription 3 (STAT3) pathway [46], which is widely expressed and activated by various growth-regulating signals and inflammatory cytokines such as interleukin-6 or interferon-γ. STAT3 plays a critical role in many biological activities, such as cell proliferation, migration, homeostasis, inflammation, immune regulation and oncogenesis [47]. In addition, STAT3 has been shown to be constitutively activated in epidermal keratinocytes of human psoriatic lesions. Therefore, inhibition of STAT3 has drastically improved clinical prognoses in psoriatic patients [48]. In contrast, miR-203 surprisingly promotes hypoproliferation in mouse skin by translationally repressing p63, ultimately inhibiting the proliferative potential of epidermal stem cells [49]. This difference alone is compelling enough to further investigate the role of miR-203 in psoriasis.

miR-146a has also been shown to be overexpressed in many psoriatic skin lesions and patients with rheumatoid arthritis [46,50]. miR-146a targets, TNF receptor-associated factor 6 (TRAF6) and IL-1R-associated kinase (IRAK) are all involved in the TNF-α pathway, which contributes to psoriatic skin inflammation. Analysis expression pattern found miR-146a to be a NF-kappaB-dependent gene [51]. Further, it has been shown that NF-kappaB activation leads to inhibition of TNF-alpha-induced apoptosis which may be regulated by miR146a overexpression, potentially contributing to the pathogenesis of psoriasis [52].

In contrast, miR-125b is downregulated in psoriasis [46] and is involved in post-transcriptional repression of TNF-α. In cases of a miR-125b downregulation, the inhibitory effect on TNF-α will be reduced, which may contribute to an increased TNF-α expression in psoriatic skin lesions. Targeting these specific miRNAs may be a promising future therapy for psoriasis.

12.8   miRNAs and wound healing

The roles of miRNAs in wound healing are not clearly defined and based on the rather sparse published data available today. However, there are several points of miRNA involvement such as apoptosis or angiogenesis, which touches on different aspects of wound healing. This will potentially be an area of interest for wound healing research in the future.

Wound healing can be divided into four phases: inflammatory, proliferative, fibroplasia and maturation, although most authors often combine the latter two steps into a remodeling phase.

After vasoconstriction and inflammation occur, platelets secrete various cytokines, including platelet-derived growth factor (PDGF), platelet factor IV and transforming growth factor beta (TGF-β). miR-140 has been shown to have a modulating effect on zebrafish PDGF receptor α [53]. Although studies on miRNA regulation of human PDGF pathways have not yet been reported, their involvement can be expected based on current efforts. miR-24 transcription has been shown to be repressed by TGF-beta1, a modulator of fibroblastic mitosis during wound healing [54].

In the proliferative phase, polymorphonuclear leukocytes and macrophages migrate to the wound site and release a variety of chemotactic factors such as fibroblast growth factor (FGF), TGF-β and

TGF-α, plasma-activated complements C3a and C5a, interleukin-1 (IL-1), tumor necrosis factor (TNF) and PDGF.

TNF-α is regulated by miR-146a targets [51], and post-transcriptional repression of TNF-α is directly targeted by miR-125b [55]. Fibroplasia, matrix deposition, angiogenesis and reepithelialization occur during the remodeling phase. At this time, fibroblasts begin to produce collagen and proteoglycans. The formation of granulation tissue is initiated together with angiogenesis, an important process during wound healing.

The role of miRNAs in angiogenesis has been the subject of numerous studies, as Dicer plays a crucial role during angiogenesis both *in vivo* and *in vitro* [56]. However, overexpression of miR-221 and miR-222 was found to indirectly reduce the expression of endothelial nitric oxide synthase (eNOS), which is essential for many endothelial cell functions [57].

In summary, miRNAs seem to be involved in the regulation of many factors influencing wound healing, raising hope for potentially new therapeutic approaches.

12.9 Perspectives and challenges

Each tissue has a specific miRNA expression profile. However to date, only a few skin-specific miRNAs have been described, and we still understand very little about their exact roles in skin physiology and pathology. We are standing at the forefront of discovery and further characterization of new miRNA pathways involved in cutaneous diseases. Current knowledge has already impacted medical and cutaneous research, and it is very likely that future efforts will continue to impact diagnostic and disease therapies. The race for diagnostic and therapeutic tools using miRNAs and the RNAi pathway has already begun for other tissues. Age-related macular degeneration and diabetic macular edema are among the first diseases treated with siRNA in clinical studies [58]. For novel miRNA-based pharmacological approaches, a variety of powerful tools are available that affect miRNA intracellular function. They include miRNA-mimetics that can replace reduced miRNAs, antagomirs that reduce overexpressed miRNAs and target protectors that enable protection of selective miRNA-binding sites [59]. Prior to implementing these potential miRNA-based therapies *in vivo*, miRNA profiling studies are necessary to further identify and characterize disease-specific miRNAs.

Profiling miRNA expression levels could lead to classification of various cancers and possibly link disease progression and prognosis to specific miRNA levels. Cancer and other immunological or infectious diseases already show certain characteristic miRNA expression patterns linked to a particular disease state [60,61]. Therefore, disease-specific miRNAs represent a potential target for disease therapy. However, several challenges should be kept in mind as future research progresses. While it is important to continue developing miRNA-based therapies, off-target effects on other cellular pathways should also be considered, particularly when a miRNA impacts expression of other physiologically relevant genes. Additional hurdles to overcome include a variety of issues in delivery, chemical stability and immune stimulation. Delivery of RNA-based therapies has previously posed a problem in the past. Although some tissues do uptake miRNAs by endocystosis, most do not. In addition, miRNAs are also susceptible to serum nucleases that cleave phosphodiester bonds between nucleotides, contributing to chemical instability. Furthermore, miRNAs are often filtered by the kidney due to their small size, which may be circumvented by complexing miRNAs to larger molecules [59]. In rapidly dividing cells, such as cancer cells, the concentration of transiently delivered miRNAs decreases faster than in slowly dividing cells, diluting out potential therapeutic activity. Viral vectors could represent an alternative to transiently delivered miRNAs depending on disease dynamics and the desired form of therapy.

The eyes, lungs and vagina have previously been shown to be easily accessible and successful targets of nucleic acid-based therapeutics. Similarly, the skin also represents an easily accessible tissue and may prove promising for local administration of therapeutic miRNAs [62].

12.10 Conclusion

Although miRNAs were initially studied in *C. elegans* and *Drosophila*, research has expanded considerably into a variety of organisms, with particularly interesting results within the field of cutaneous biology. Further investigation of miRNA function and its impact on cutaneous physiology and pathology will change our understanding of gene regulation in the skin. Elucidation of new miRNA pathways involved in skin development and skin pathology will undoubtedly lead us into a new era of miRNA-based pharmacological therapies.

12.11 References

1) Levy S, Sutton G, Ng PC et al.: The diploid genome sequence of an individual human. PLoS Biol 5: e254,2007.

2) van der Krol AR, Mur LA, Beld M, Mol JN, Stuitje AR: Flavonoid genes in petunia: addition of a limited number of gene copies may lead to a suppression of gene expression. Plant Cell 2: 291 299,1990.

3) Fire A, Xu S, Montgomery MK, Kostas SA, Driver SE, Mello CC: Potent and specific genetic interference by double-stranded RNA in Caenorhabditis elegans. Nature 391: 806 811,1998.

4) Montgomery MK, Xu S, Fire A: RNA as target of double-stranded RNA-mediated genetic interference in Caenorhabditis elegans. Proc Natl Acad Sci 95: 15502 15507,1998.

5) Elbashir SM, Harborth J, Lendeckel W, Yalcin A, Weber K, Tuschl T: Duplexes of 21-nucleotide RNAs mediate RNA interference in cultured mammalian cells. Nature 411: 494 498,2001.

6) Parrish S, Fleenor J, Xu S, Mello C, Fire A: Functional anatomy of a dsRNA trigger: Differential requirements for the two trigger strands in RNA interference. Molec Cell 6: 1077 1087,2000.

7) Lee RC, Feinbaum RL, Ambros V: The C elegans heterochronic gene lin-4 encodes small RNAs with antisense complementarity to lin-14. Cell 75:843 854,1993.

8) Reinhart BJ, Slack FJ, Basson M et al.: The 21-nucleotide let-7 RNA regulates developmental timing in Caenorhabditis elegans. Nature 403: 901 906,2000.

9) Grishok A, Pasquinelli AE, Conte D et al.: Genes and mechanisms related to RNA interference regulate expression of the small temporal RNAs that control C. elegans developmental timing. Cell 106: 23 34,2001.

10) Ambros V, Bartel B, Bartel DP et al.: A uniform system for microRNA annotation. RNA 9: 277 279,2003.

11) Bartel DP: MicroRNAs: genomics, biogenesis, mechanism, and function. Cell 116: 281 297,2004.

12) Lin SL, Miller JD, Ying SY: Intronic MicroRNA (miRNA). J Biomed Biotechnol 4: 26818,2006.

13) Lee Y, Jeon K, Lee JT, Kim S, Kim VN: MicroRNA maturation: stepwise processing and subcellular localization. EMBO J 21: 4663 4670,2002.

14) Lee Y, Ahn C, Han J, Choi H, Kim J, Yim J, Lee J, Provost P, Rådmark O, Kim S, Kim VN: The nuclear RNase III Drosha initiates microRNA processing. Nature 425: 415 419,2003.

15) Han J, Lee Y, Yeom KH, Kim YK, Jin H, Kim VN. The Drosha-DGCR8 complex in primary microRNA processing. Genes Dev 18: 3016 3027,2004.

16) Landthaler M, Yalcin A, Tuschl T: LaThe human DiGeorge syndrome critical region gene 8 and Its D. melanogaster homolog are required for miRNA biogenesis. Curr Biol 14: 2162 2167,2004.

17) Bohnsack MT, Czaplinski K, Gorlich D: Exportin 5 is a RanGTP-dependent dsRNA-binding protein that mediates nuclear export of pre-miRNAs. RNA 10: 185 191,2004.

18) Yi R, Qin Y, Macara IG, Cullen BR: Exportin-5 mediates the nuclear export of pre-microRNAs and short hairpin RNAs. Genes Dev 17: 3011 3016,2003.

19) Lee Y, Hur I, Park SY, Kim YK, Suh MR, Kim VN: The role of PACT in the RNA silencing pathway. EMBO J 25: 522 532,2006.

20) Song JJ, Liu J, Tolia NH, Schneiderman J, Smith SK, Martienssen RA, Hannon GJ, Joshua-Tor L: The crystal structure of the Argonaute2 PAZ domain reveals an RNA binding motif in RNAi effector complexes. Nat Struct Biol 10: 1026 1032,2003.

21) Dalmay T: MicroRNAs and cancer. J Intern Med 263: 366 375,2008.

22) Griffiths-Jones S, Saini HK, van Dongen S, Enright AJ: miRBase: tools for microRNA genomics. Nucleic Acids Res 36:154 158,2008.

23) Yi R, O'Carroll D, Pasolli HA, Zhang Z, Dietrich FS, Tarakhovsky A, Fuchs E: Morphogenesis in skin is governed by discrete sets of differentially expressed microRNAs. Nat Genet 38: 356 362,2006.

24) Andl T, Murchison EP, Liu F et al.: The miRNA-processing enzyme dicer is essential for the morphogenesis and maintenance of hair follicles. Curr Biol 16: 1041 1049,2006.

25) Yi R, Poy MN, Stoffel M, Fuchs E: A skin microRNA promotes differentiation by repressing 'stemness'. Nature 452: 225 229,2008.

26) Koster MI, Kim S, Mills AA, DeMayo FJ, Roop DR: p63 is the molecular switch for initiation of an epithelial stratification program. Genes Dev 18: 126 131,2004.

27) McKeon F: p63 and the epithelial stem cell: more than status quo? Genes Dev 18: 465 469,2004.

28) McClure LV, Sullivan CS: Kaposi's sarcoma herpes virus taps into a host microRNA regulatory network. Cell Host Microbe 3: 1 3,2008.

29) Zhang L, Huang J, Yang N et al.: microRNAs exhibit high frequency genomic alterations in human cancer. Proc Natl Acad Sci USA 103: 9136 9141,2006.

30) Gaur A, Jewell DA, Liang Y, Ridzon D, Moore JH, Chen C, Ambros VR, Israel MA: Characterization of and their biological correlates in human cancer cell lines. Cancer Res 67: 2456 2468,2007.

31) Bemis LT, Chen R, Amato CM, Classen EH, Robinson SE, Coffey DG, Erickson PF, Shellman YG, Robinson WA: MicroRNA-137 targets microphthalmia-associated transcription factor in melanoma cell lines. Cancer Res 68: 1362 1368,2008.

32) Cui R, Widlund HR, Feige E, Lin JY, Wilensky DL, Igras VE, D'Orazio J, Fung CY, Schanbacher CF, Granter SR, Fisher DE: Central role of p53 in the suntan response and pathologic hyperpigmentation. Cell 128: 853 864,2007.

33) Dynek JN, Chan SM, Liu J, Zha J, Fairbrother WJ, Vucic D: Microphthalmia-associated transcription factor is a critical transcriptional regulator of melanoma inhibitor of apoptosis in melanomas. Cancer Res 68: 3124 3132,2008.

34) Felicetti F, Errico MC, Bottero L et al.: The promyelocytic leukemia zinc finger-microRNA-221/-222 pathway controls melanoma progression through multiple oncogenic mechanisms: Cancer Res 68: 2745 2754,2008.

35) Alexeev V, Yoon K: Distinctive role of the cKit receptor tyrosine kinase signaling in mammalian melanocytes. J Invest Dermatol 126: 1102 1110,2006.

36) Felicetti F, Bottero L, Felli N, Mattia G, Labbaye C, Alvino E, Peschle C, Colombo MP, Carè A: Role of PLZF in melanoma progression. Oncogene 23: 4567 4576,2004.

37) Schultz J, Lorenz P, Gross G, Ibrahim S, Kunz M: MicroRNA let-7b targets important cell cycle molecules in malignant melanoma cells and interferes with anchorage-independent growth. Cell Res 18: 549 557,2008.

38) Worley LA, Long MD, Onken MD, Harbour JW: Micro-RNAs associated with metastasis in uveal melanoma identified by multiplexed microarray profiling. Melanoma Res 18: 184 190,2008.

39) Molnár V, Tamási V, Bakos B, Wiener Z, Falus A: Changes in miRNA expression in solid tumors: an miRNA profiling in melanomas. Semin Cancer Biol 18: 111 122,2008.

40) Skalsky RL, Samols MA, Plaisance KB: Kaposi's sarcoma-associated herpesvirus encodes an ortholog of miR-155. J Virol 81: 12836 12845,2007.

41) Gottwein E, Cai X, Cullen BR: A novel assay for viral microRNA function identifies a single nucleotide polymorphism that affects Drosha processing. J Virol 80: 5321 5326,2006.

42) Tam W, Ben-Yehuda D, Hayward WS: bic, a novel gene activated by proviral insertions in avian leukosis virus-induced lymphomas, is likely to function through its noncoding RNA. Mol Cell Biol 17: 1490 1502,1997.

43) Ettehadi P, Greaves MW, Wallach D, Aderka D, Camp RD: Elevated tumour necrosis factor-alpha (TNF-alpha) biological activity in psoriatic skin lesions. Clin Exp Immunol 96: 146 151,1994.

44) Sonkoly E, Ståhle M, Pivarcsi A. MicroRNAs and immunity: novel players in the regulation of normal immune function and inflammation. Semin Cancer Biol 18: 131 140,2008.

45) Chen CZ, Li L, Lodish HF et al.: MicroRNAs modulate hematopoietic lineage differentiation. Science 303: 83 86,2004.

46) Sonkoly E, Ståhle M, Pivarcsi A: MicroRNAs: novel regulators in skin inflammation. Clin Exp Dermatol 33: 312-315,2008.

47) Aaronson DS, Horvath CM: A road map for those who don't know JAK-STAT. Science 296: 1653 1655,2002.

48) Sano S, Chan KS, DiGiovanni J: Impact of Stat3 activation upon skin biology: a dichotomy of its role between homeostasis and diseases. J Dermatol Sci 50: 1 14,2008.

49) Koster MI, Dai D, Marinari B et al.: p63 induces key target genes required for epidermal morphogenesis. Proc Natl Acad Sci USA 104: 3255 3260,2007.

50) Pauley KM, Satoh M, Chan AL: Upregulated miR-146a expression in peripheral blood mononuclear cells from rheumatoid arthritis patients. Arthritis Res Ther 10: R101,2008.

51) Taganov KD, Boldin MP, Chang KJ et al.: NF-kappaB-dependent induction of microRNA miR-146, an inhibitor targeted to signaling proteins of innate immune responses. Proc Natl Acad Sci USA 103: 12481 12486,2006.

52) Tang G, Minemoto Y, Dibling B: Inhibition of JNK activation through NF-kappaB target genes. Nature 414: 313 317,2001.

53) Eberhart JK, He X, Swartz ME et al.: MicroRNA Mirn140 modulates Pdgf signaling during palatogenesis. Nat Genet 40: 290 298,2008.

54) Sun Q, Zhang Y, Yang G et al.: Transforming growth factor-beta-regulated miR-24 promotes skeletal muscle differentiation. Nucleic Acids Res 36: 2690 2699,2008.

55) Tili E, Michaille JJ, Cimino A et al.: Modulation of miR-155 and miR-125b levels following lipopolysaccharide/TNF-alpha stimulation and their possible roles in regulating the response to endotoxin shock. J Immunol 179: 5082 5089,2007.

56) Kuehbacher A, Urbich C, Dimmeler S: Targeting microRNA expression to regulate angiogenesis. Trends Pharmacol Sci 29: 12 15,2008.

57) Suárez Y, Fernández-Hernando C, Pober JS, Sessa WC: Dicer dependent microRNAs regulate gene expression and functions in human endothelial cells. Circ Res 100: 1164 1173,2007.

58) http://clinicaltrials.gov (ClinicalTrials.gov Identifier: NCT00306904 and NCT00363714)

59) Love TM, Moffett HF, Novina CD.Not miR-ly small RNAs: big potential for microRNAs in therapy. J Allergy Clin Immunol 121: 309 319,2008.

60) Wang M, Tan LP, Dijkstra MK et al.: miRNA analysis in B-cell chronic lymphocytic leukaemia: proliferation centres characterized by low miR-150 and high BIC/miR-155 expression. J Pathol: 215: 13 20,2008.

61) Marton S, Garcia MR, Robello C et al.: Small RNAs analysis in CLL reveals a deregulation of miRNA expression and novel miRNA candidates of putative relevance in CLL pathogenesis. Leukemia 22: 330 338,2008.

62) Soifer HS, Rossi JJ, Saetrom P. MicroRNAs in disease and potential therapeutic applications. Mol Ther 15: 2070-9,2007.

63) Chen CZ. MicroRNAs as oncogenes and tumor suppressors. N Engl J Med 353: 1768 1771,2005.

13 Paper 9: microRNA in non-melanoma skin cancer*

13.1 Introduction

MicroRNAs (miRNAs) are 17- to 23-nucleotide (nt), short, non-coding RNA molecules that are capable of regulating gene expression at a post-transcriptional level. Encoded within both exons and introns, they play a pivotal role in a variety of physiologic cellular functions and diseases, including cancer. Approximately 30%–60% of all human genes are affected by miRNA regulation, and our understanding of their role as both tumor suppressors and oncogenes in a variety of different cancers is gradually evolving. In this mini-review, we summarize the current knowledge on the role of miRNAs in non-melanoma skin cancer (NMSC). All the differentially expressed miRNAs in NMSC have been compiled in table 12-1.

13.2 miRNA maturation and function

Briefly, miRNA maturation begins in the nucleus where RNA polymerase II transcribes the primary-miRNA (pri-miRNA) transcript. Drosha, an intranuclear RNase III endonuclease, and its co-factor, DiGeorge syndrome critical region gene 8 (DGCR8 or Pasha (Partner of Drosha)), form the microprocessor complex that cleaves the pri-miRNA transcript into several 70–90-nt precursor-miRNAs (pre-miRNAs) that share a characteristic stem loop structure [1]. These pre-miRNAs are transported from the nucleus to the cytoplasm by exportin-5 (Exp-5). In the cytoplasm, Dicer, an extranuclear RNase III enzyme, cuts the pre-miRNAs into mature miRNA strands, that are loaded into the RNA-induced silencing complex (RISC).

Depending on the degree of complementarity between the target mRNA and the miRNA, binding either stops translation by cleaving the target mRNA (full complementarity) or suppresses translation by binding to and impeding ribosomal reading of the mRNA (incomplete complementarity).

---

* Co-authors: Daniel Sand M.D., Peter Altmeyer M.D., Falk G. Bechara M.D.

Tab. 13-1: Listing selected microRNAs (miRNAs) and their molecular impact relevant to non-melanoma skin cancer (n.a.=not available)

miRNA	Regulation	Tumor	Molecular Impact	Author miRNA	Author Molecular Impact
let-7	+	BCC	involved in regulating cell proliferation	Heffelfinger et al.[12]	Heffelfinger et al.[12]
hsa-miR-17	+	BCC	pro-growth miRNA regulated in vitro by MAPK/ERK-induced phosphorylation of TRBP	Sand et al.[13]	Parroo et al. [29]
hsa-miR-18a	+	BCC	member of the hsa-miR-17-92 cluster, also known as Oncomir-1; responsible for enhanced cell proliferation and the suppression of apoptosis	Sand et al.[13]	He et al.[30] Al-Nakhle et al.[31]
hsa-miR-18b	+	BCC	same seed sequence as hsa-miR-18a	Sand et al.[13]	
hsa-miR-19b	+	BCC	member of the hsa-miR-17-92 cluster, also known as Oncomir-1; responsible for enhanced cell proliferation and the suppression of apoptosis	Sand et al.[13]	He et al.[30] Al-Nakhle et al.[31]
hsa-miR-19b-1*	+	BCC	member of the hsa-miR-17-92 cluster, also known as Oncomir-1; responsible for enhanced cell proliferation and the suppression of apoptosis	Sand et al.[13]	He et al.[30] Al-Nakhle et al.[31]

Tab. 13-1: (Continued)

miRNA	Regulation	Tumor	Molecular Impact	Author miRNA	Author Molecular Impact
hsa-miR-21	+ +	BCC SCC	UVA radiation results in increased expression; oncogene that represses a variety of tumor suppressors such as PTEN and PCDC4	Heffelfinger et al.[12] Dziunycz et al.[23]	Heffelfinger et al.[12]
hsa-miR-29c	-	BCC	associated with hypermethylation of tumor-related genes and disease outcome in cutaneous melanoma; downregulates DNA methyltransferases DNMT3A and DNMT3B	Sand et al.[13]	Nguyen et al. [32]
hsa-miR-29c*	-	BCC	n.a.	Sand et al.[13]	
hsa-miR-93	+	BCC	part of the hsa-miR-106b-25 cluster; transcription factor E2F1 is a target gene of hsa-miR-93	Sand et al.[13]	Li et al.[33]
hsa-miR-106b	+	BCC	part of the hsa-miR-106b-25; transcription factor E2F1 is a target gene of hsa-miR-106b	Sand et al.[13]	Li et al.[33]
hsa-miR-124	-	SCC	correlates inversely with tumor progression, regulates ERK2 together with hsa-miR-214	Yamane et al.[24]	Yamane et al.[24]

Tab. 13-1: (Continued)

miRNA	Regulation	Tumor	Molecular Impact	Author miRNA	Author Molecular Impact
hsa-miR-125a-5p	+	BCC	induces apoptosis via a p53-dependent pathway (shown in human lung cancer cells)	Sand et al.[13]	Jiang et al. [34]
hsa-miR-130a	+	BCC	predicted regulatory effect on the apoptosis regulator BCL-2	Sand et al.[13]	Sand et al.[13]
hsa-miR-139-5p	-	BCC	n.a.	Sand et al.[13]	
hsa-miR-140-3p	-	BCC	n.a.	Sand et al.[13]	
hsa-miR-143	+	BCC	n.a.	Heffelfinger et al.[12]	
hsa-miR-145	-	BCC	targets epidermal growth factor receptor (EGFR) and nucleoside diphosphate linked moiety X-type motif 1 (NUDT1) (shown in lung adenocarcinoma)	Sand et al.[13]	Cho et al.[35]
hsa-miR-148a	+	BCC	n.a.	Heffelfinger et al.[12]	

Tab. 13-1: (Continued)

miRNA	Regulation	Tumor	Molecular Impact	Author miRNA	Author Molecular Impact
hsa-miR-181c	+	BCC	targets NOTCH4 and KRAS which have both been implicated in the pathogenesis of BCC	Sand et al.[13]	Proweller at al.[36] van der Schroeff et al.[37]
hsa-miR-181c*	+	BCC	n.a.	Sand et al.[13]	
hsa-miR-181d	+	BCC	n.a.	Sand et al.[13]	
hsa-miR-182	+	BCC	described to negatively regulate human Forkhead-box O1 (FOXO1) and linked to oncogenic transformation	Heffelfinger et al.[12] Sand et al.[13]	Guttilla et al.[38]
hsa-miR-184	+	SCC		Dziunycz et al.[23]	
hsa-miR-214	-	SCC	correlates inversely with tumor progression, regulates ERK1	Yamane et al.[24]	Yamane et al.[24]
hsa-miR-378	+	BCC	n.a.	Heffelfinger et al.[12]	

The miRNA multiprotein effector RISC is composed of the following components: argonaute-1 (AGO1, eukaryotic translation initiation factor 2C.1, EIF2C1), argonaute-2 (AGO2, eukaryotic translation initiation factor 2C.2, EIF2C2), the double-stranded RNA-binding protein (dsRBP) activator of protein kinase R (PACT), Dicer-substrate complex stabilizing methyltransferase TAR HIV-1 RNA binding protein 1 (TARBP1), RISC-loading complex subunit TAR HIV-1 RNA binding protein 2 (TARBP2), metadherin [MTDH, also known as protein LYRIC or astrocyte elevated gene-1 protein (AEG-1)], and staphylococcal nuclease and tudor domain containing 1 (SND1) [2-5].

13.3   miRNA in basal cell carcinoma

Basal cell carcinoma (BCC) is the most common form of human cancer [6]. Although it rarely metastasizes (1:50,000), it has a huge socioeconomic impact on healthcare systems worldwide because of its high incidence [7].

In some cases, when diagnosed late or neglected by the patient, the growing horizontal and vertical extension of BCC can lead to disfigurement or complications including the death of the patient in cases in which vital structures are affected. In advanced cases, tumor growth can spread to types of tissue other than skin, such as cartilage, bone, nerves, and vessels [8].

The potential role of miRNA dysregulation in BCC development has recently started to develop as a new path to enlighten the pathology of BCC. The miRNA machinery components including the microprocessor complex consisting of Drosha, DGCR8, Dicer, and the RISC components argonaute-1, argonaute-2, PACT, TARBP1 and TARBP2 have recently been investigated regarding their expression in both BCC and cSCC [9, 10]. The Drosha, DGCR8, AGO1, AGO2, PACT, and TARBP1 expression levels have been shown to be significantly higher in BCC and cutaneous squamous cell carcinoma (cSCC) when compared to healthy controls [10]. While this initial screening of the miRNA machinery in BCC was the first study that searched for the possible role of miRNA involvement in BCC pathogenesis, the focus has now shifted toward more specific miRNA profiling studies.

Although not peer-reviewed, Lovén was the first to describe a genome-wide analysis of miRNA expression in human healthy skin and BCC as a part of a doctoral thesis [11]. Lovén demonstrated that hsa-mir-203 shows a ~5-fold decrease in BCC and that hsa-miR-203 was expressed in the suprabasal layers of healthy skin, while BCCs consistently lacked hsa-miR-203 expression as claimed to be shown by *in situ* hybridization with specific locked nucleic acid probes. Furthermore, the author describes the significant negative correlation between hsa-miR-203 expression and *GLI1*, a transcription factor that mediates the hedgehog pathway, as well as protein patched homolog 1 (*PTCH1*), the sonic hedgehog receptor, indicating that a loss of hsa-miR-203 may be associated with aberrant hedgehog signaling in BCC. Heffelfinger et al. were the first to publish peer-reviewed data regarding miRNA expression profiles in BCC [12]. In their recent genome sequencing study, they investigated eight nodular and eight infiltrative BCCs and were able to show that hsa-miR-21, hsa-miR-143, hsa-miR-148a, hsa-miR-378, hsa-miR-182, and hsa-let-7 family members were the most highly expressed. Additionally, they described 21 miRNAs that showed a statistically significant difference in expression between nodular and infiltrative BCCs. A microarray-based miRNA profiling studies of BCC has recently identified sixteen significantly up-regulated (hsa-miR-17, miR-18a, hsa-miR-18b, hsa-miR-19b, hsa-miR-19b-1*, hsa-miR-93, hsa-miR-106b, hsa-miR-125a-5p, hsa-miR-130a, hsa-miR-181c, hsa-miR-181c*, hsa-miR-181d, hsa-miR-182, hsa-miR-455-3p, hsa-miR-455-5p and hsa-miR-542-5p) and ten significantly down-regulated (hsa-miR-29c, hsa-miR-29c*, hsa-miR-139-5p, hsa-miR-140-3p, hsa-miR-145, hsa-miR-378, hsa-miR-572, hsa-miR-638, hsa-miR-2861 and hsa-miR-3196) miRNAs in BCC compared with non-lesional skin. Data mining revealed connections to tumor-promoting pathways, such as the hedgehog and the MAPK/ERK signaling cascades which have previously been connected to BCC [13]. Although the latter studies are descriptive, based on these results, skin cancer scientists will be able to further investigate the possible role of specific miRNAs in functional studies.

13.4   miRNA in cutaneous squamous cell carcinoma

cSCC is an epithelial skin tumor that is the second most common form of human cancer [6]. Depending on the depth of the lesions, it can result in metastasis with fatal consequences accounting for 20% of all skin cancer-related deaths [14, 15]. Some cSCCs become locally invasive and show an aggressive course [16]. The rate of metastasis has been shown to be 0.3–3.7% with an overall 5-year survival rate <30% in cases in which it spreads systemically [17].

The role of miRNAs in SCC of different origins has been investigated in cervical, lung, esophageal, oral, pharyngeal, and tongue tissue [18-22]. Investigations of the involvement of miRNA dysregulation in cSCC have just recently begun. Similar to BCC, the expression levels of the miRNA machinery, namely Drosha, DGCR8, AGO1, AGO2, PACT, and TARBP1, were significantly higher compared to healthy controls and Dicer levels were significantly higher compared to intra-individual controls [9, 10]. Furthermore, Dziunycz et al. have investigated a distinct set of miRNAs (hsa-miR-21, hsa-miR-203, hsa-miR-205, and hsa-miR-184) in cSCC modulated by UV radiation [23]. They described the significantly increased expression of hsa-miR-21 and hsa-miR-184 and the decreased expression of hsa-miR-203 in cSCC. Interestingly, they found that UVA increased the expression of hsa-miR-21, hsa-miR-203, and hsa-miR-205, whereas UVB increased hsa-miR-203 and decreased hsa-miR-205.

Yamane et al. showed that hsa-miR-214 is the regulator of extracellular-signal-regulated kinase 1 (ERK1 or – mitogen-activated protein kinase 3 MAPK3) and hsa-miR-124 and hsa-miR-214 are both regulators of ERK2 (mitogen-activated protein kinase 1 or MAPK1) [24]. Both, hsa-miR-124 and hsa-miR-214, were shown to be significantly down-regulated in SCC in vitro and in vivo.

As human-papilloma-virus (HPV) has been associated with the development of NMSC, it is interesting to note that a study by Gu et al. was the first to associate miRNA let-7a expression with HPV-38 infection [25]. HPV-38 infection has recently shown to significantly contribute to cSCC development rendering keratinocytes more susceptible to UV-induced carcinogenesis in a transgenic mouse model [26]. Whether other cSCC associated HPVs show any miRNA dysregulation needs to be investigated in the future.

13.5 Conclusion

Although the role of miRNAs in NMSC is just beginning to be understood, the early results have shown preliminary evidence that miRNAs are involved in the pathology of NMSC. The following points needs to be discussed, as we believe that they are essential for improving further miRNA research in NMSC.

1) The studies that are available to date were performed with tissue of skin biopsies that consist of dermal and epidermal tissue. We believe that data quality can be increased by using laser microdissected tumor material, as the specificity of the findings would increase. Our initial experience with laser microdissection in melanoma tissue has shown that the RNA quality of laser microdissected, cryofixed tissue is often too poor to be considered for further studies; however, this may not necessarily be the case for paraffin-embedded NMSC tissue. We therefore believe that it would be desirable to use laser microdissected paraffin-embedded NMSC tissue when possible.

2) The studies that are available are based on very small sample sizes (n<10), and in terms of data quality, it would be beneficial to expand the sample size.

3) Functional studies involving antagomirs are highly desirable, as they could confirm descriptive studies and pave the way for alternative, miRNA-based forms of therapy in the future [27, 28].

13.6 References

[1]   Sand M, Gambichler T, Sand D, Skrygan M, Altmeyer P,
        Bechara FG. MicroRNAs and the skin: tiny players in the body's
        largest organ. J Dermatol Sci. 2009;53; 169-175.

[2]   Emdad L, Sarkar D, Su ZZ, Randolph A, Boukerche H, Valerie
        K, et al. Activation of the nuclear factor kappaB pathway by
        astrocyte elevated gene-1: implications for tumor progression
        and metastasis. Cancer Res. 2006;66; 1509-1516.

[3]   Lee Y, Hur I, Park SY, Kim YK, Suh MR, Kim VN. The role of
        PACT in the RNA silencing pathway. EMBO J. 2006;25; 522-
        532.

[4]   Caudy AA, Ketting RF, Hammond SM, Denli AM, Bathoorn AM,
        Tops BB, et al. A micrococcal nuclease homologue in RNAi
        effector complexes. Nature. 2003;425; 411-414.

[5]   Yoo BK, Santhekadur PK, Gredler R, Chen D, Emdad L, Bhutia
        S, et al. Increased RNA-induced silencing complex (RISC)
        activity contributes to hepatocellular carcinoma. Hepatology.
        2011;53; 1538-1548.

[6]   Ratushny V, Gober MD, Hick R, Ridky TW, Seykora JT. From
        keratinocyte to cancer: the pathogenesis and modeling of
        cutaneous squamous cell carcinoma. J Clin Invest. 2012;122;
        464-472.

[7]   Jung GW, Metelitsa AI, Dover DC, Salopek TG. Trends in
        incidence of nonmelanoma skin cancers in Alberta, Canada,
        1988-2007. Br J Dermatol. 2010;163; 146-154.

[8]   Jarus-Dziedzic K, Zub W, Dziedzic D, Jelen M, Krotochwil J,
        Mierzejewski M. Multiple metastases of carcinoma basocellulare
        into spinal column. J Neurooncol. 2000;48; 57-62.

[9]   Sand M, Gambichler T, Skrygan M, Sand D, Scola N, Altmeyer
        P, et al. Expression levels of the microRNA processing enzymes
        Drosha and dicer in epithelial skin cancer. Cancer Invest.
        2010;28; 649-653.

[10] Sand M, Skrygan M, Georgas D, Arenz C, Gambichler T, Sand D, et al. Expression levels of the microRNA maturing microprocessor complex component DGCR8 and the RNA-induced silencing complex (RISC) components Argonaute-1, Argonaute-2, PACT, TARBP1, and TARBP2 in epithelial skin cancer. Mol Carcinog. 2011.

[11] Lovén J. Functional studies of microRNAs in development and cancer; 2010; Department of Microbiology, Tumor and Cell Biology Karolinska Institutet, Stockholm, Sweden; http://diss.kib. ki.se/2010/978-91-7457-031-1/thesis.pdf.

[12] Heffelfinger C, Ouyang Z, Engberg A, Leffell DJ, Hanlon AM, Gordon PB, et al. Correlation of Global MicroRNA Expression With Basal Cell Carcinoma Subtype. G3 (Bethesda). 2012;2; 279-286.

[13] Sand M, Skrygan M, Sand D, Georgas D, Hahn S, Gambichler T, et al. Expression of microRNAs in basal cell carcinoma. Br J Dermatol. 2012.

[14] Rowe DE, Carroll RJ, Day CL, Jr. Prognostic factors for local recurrence, metastasis, and survival rates in squamous cell carcinoma of the skin, ear, and lip. Implications for treatment modality selection. J Am Acad Dermatol. 1992;26; 976-990.

[15] Mohle J, Nickoloff BJ. Fatal cutaneous squamous cell carcinoma in a forty-three-year-old male. J Dermatol Surg Oncol. 1986;12; 276-279.

[16] Cassarino DS, Derienzo DP, Barr RJ. Cutaneous squamous cell carcinoma: a comprehensive clinicopathologic classification. Part one. J Cutan Pathol. 2006;33; 191-206.

[17] Kwa RE, Campana K, Moy RL. Biology of cutaneous squamous cell carcinoma. J Am Acad Dermatol. 1992;26; 1-26.

[18] Muralidhar B, Winder D, Murray M, Palmer R, Barbosa-Morais N, Saini H, et al. Functional evidence that Drosha overexpression in cervical squamous cell carcinoma affects cell phenotype and microRNA profiles. J Pathol. 2011;224; 496-507.

[19] Yang Y, Li X, Yang Q, Wang X, Zhou Y, Jiang T, et al. The role of microRNA in human lung squamous cell carcinoma. Cancer Genet Cytogenet. 2010;200; 127-133.

[20]   Mathe EA, Nguyen GH, Bowman ED, Zhao Y, Budhu A, Schetter AJ, et al. MicroRNA expression in squamous cell carcinoma and adenocarcinoma of the esophagus: associations with survival. Clin Cancer Res. 2009;15; 6192-6200.

[21]   Lajer CB, Nielsen FC, Friis-Hansen L, Norrild B, Borup R, Garnaes E, et al. Different miRNA signatures of oral and pharyngeal squamous cell carcinomas: a prospective translational study. Br J Cancer. 2011;104; 830-840.

[22]   Li J, Huang H, Sun L, Yang M, Pan C, Chen W, et al. MiR-21 indicates poor prognosis in tongue squamous cell carcinomas as an apoptosis inhibitor. Clin Cancer Res. 2009;15; 3998-4008.

[23]   Dziunycz P, Iotzova-Weiss G, Eloranta JJ, Lauchli S, Hafner J, French LE, et al. Squamous cell carcinoma of the skin shows a distinct microRNA profile modulated by UV radiation. J Invest Dermatol. 2010;130; 2686-2689.

[24]   Yamane K, Jinnin M, Etoh T, Kobayashi Y, Shimozono N, Fukushima S, et al. Down-regulation of miR-124/-214 in cutaneous squamous cell carcinoma mediates abnormal cell proliferation via the induction of ERK. J Mol Med (Berl). 2012.

[25]   Gu W, An J, Ye P, Zhao KN, Antonsson A. Prediction of conserved microRNAs from skin and mucosal human papillomaviruses. Arch Virol. 2011;156; 1161-1171.

[26]   Viarisio D, Mueller-Decker K, Kloz U, Aengeneyndt B, Kopp-Schneider A, Grone HJ, et al. E6 and E7 from beta HPV38 cooperate with ultraviolet light in the development of actinic keratosis-like lesions and squamous cell carcinoma in mice. PLoS Pathog. 2011;7; e1002125.

[27]   Czech MP. MicroRNAs as therapeutic targets. N Engl J Med. 2006;354; 1194-1195.

[28]   Krutzfeldt J, Rajewsky N, Braich R, Rajeev KG, Tuschl T, Manoharan M, et al. Silencing of microRNAs in vivo with 'antagomirs'. Nature. 2005;438; 685-689.

[29]   Paroo Z, Ye X, Chen S, Liu Q. Phosphorylation of the human microRNA-generating complex mediates MAPK/Erk signaling. Cell. 2009;139; 112-122.

[30]   He L, Thomson JM, Hemann MT, Hernando-Monge E, Mu D, Goodson S, et al. A microRNA polycistron as a potential human oncogene. Nature. 2005;435; 828-833.

[31]   Al-Nakhle H, Burns PA, Cummings M, Hanby AM, Hughes TA, Satheesha S, et al. Estrogen receptor {beta}1 expression is regulated by miR-92 in breast cancer. Cancer Res. 2010;70; 4778-4784.

[32]   Nguyen T, Kuo C, Nicholl MB, Sim MS, Turner RR, Morton DL, et al. Downregulation of microRNA-29c is associated with hypermethylation of tumor-related genes and disease outcome in cutaneous melanoma. Epigenetics. 2011;6; 388-394.

[33]   Li Y, Tan W, Neo TW, Aung MO, Wasser S, Lim SG, et al. Role of the miR-106b-25 microRNA cluster in hepatocellular carcinoma. Cancer Sci. 2009;100; 1234-1242.

[34]   Jiang LH, Q.; Chang, J.; Wang, E.; Qiu, X. MicroRNA HSA-miR-125a-5p induces apoptosis by activating p53 in lung cancer cells. Exp Lung Res.2011 Sep;37(7):387-98.

[35]   Cho WC, Chow AS, Au JS. MiR-145 inhibits cell proliferation of human lung adenocarcinoma by targeting EGFR and NUDT1. RNA Biol. 2011;8; 125-131.

[36]   Proweller A, Tu L, Lepore JJ, Cheng L, Lu MM, Seykora J, et al. Impaired notch signaling promotes de novo squamous cell carcinoma formation. Cancer Res. 2006;66; 7438-7444.

[37]   van der Schroeff JG, Evers LM, Boot AJ, Bos JL. Ras oncogene mutations in basal cell carcinomas and squamous cell carcinomas of human skin. J Invest Dermatol. 1990;94; 423-425.

[38]   Guttilla IK, White BA. Coordinate regulation of FOXO1 by miR-27a, miR-96, and miR-182 in breast cancer cells. J Biol Chem. 2009;284; 23204-23216.